# PRAISE FOR *MISDIAGNOSED*

"So many people who come to Amen Clinics have been misdiagnosed and it has nearly ruined their lives. Jody Berger's new book, *Misdiagnosed*, is a thoughtful, powerful story about a journey from desperation to hope and then healing. I highly recommend it."

—Daniel G. Amen, MD, author of *Change Your Brain, Change Your Life*

"In this compelling, beautifully written book, Jody Berger offers an empowering look at the many flaws in our medical system and brings home the importance of both trusting your own knowledge in seeking diagnosis and treatment as well as finding the strength and confidence to take charge of your health and partner with the right practitioners."

—Mary Shomon, *New York Times* bestselling author and patient advocate

"Jody Berger movingly details her exhausting but ultimately triumphant journey to healing after a diagnosis of MS. Her indefatigable quest to find the right doctor and the right cure underscores the fact that there is no such thing as one size fits all in medicine."

—Gayatri Devi, MD, clinical associate professor, NYU School of Medicine, and author of *A Calm Brain*

# *Misdiagnosed*

## ONE WOMAN'S TOUR OF —AND ESCAPE FROM— HEALTHCARELAND

JODY BERGER

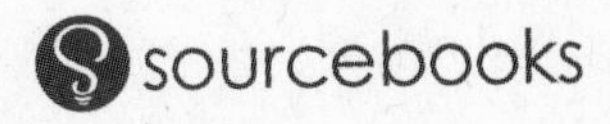

This book is not intended as a substitute for medical advice from a qualified physician. The intent of this book is to provide accurate general information in regard to the subject matter covered. If medical advice or other expert help is needed, the services of an appropriate medical professional should be sought.

This book is a memoir. It reflects the author's present recollections of her experiences over a period of years. Some names and characteristics have been changed, some events have been compressed, and some dialogue has been re-created.



Published by Sourcebooks, Inc.
P.O. Box 4410, Naperville, Illinois 60567-4410
(630) 961-3900
Fax: (630) 961-2168
www.sourcebooks.com

Library of Congress Cataloging-in-Publication Data

Berger, Jody.
Misdiagnosed : one woman's tour of and escape from healthcareland / Jody Berger.
pages cm
1. Berger, Jody—Health. 2. Celiac disease—Patients—United States—Biography. 3. Celiac disease—Diagnosis—United States. 4. Medical errors—United States. I. Title.
RC862.C44B47 2014
616.3'99—dc23

2014018555

Printed and bound in the United States of America.
VP 10 9 8 7 6 5 4 3 2 1

# CONTENTS

## CHAPTER 1

# EVERYTHING IN MODERATION

I had never been in the hospital before. Not for myself, anyway. I'd never broken a bone, had a tonsil removed or been that sick. I'd only gone to the hospital for others. When my sister had her sons, I went, and years later, when a friend had surgery, I brought a plant to set on the windowsill in his sunny, white room.

The only other time I went to a hospital was when I was on assignment. The newspaper I worked for sent me to Canada in hopes of getting a quote from an injured hockey player. He didn't want to talk. In case he changed his mind, though, I sat in the waiting room day after day. It didn't seem so bad. Boring maybe, but not scary.

This time was different. This trip was supposedly for me, for a test to tell me what was wrong with *me*. I'd just flown home from Christmas with my cousins and had a few days to collect last-minute things before flying to India on New Year's Day. I told myself it was no big deal, that going to the hospital and getting an MRI was just another item on my to-do list, right after buying bug spray.

I circled the hospital buildings and found a spot among the acres and acres of parked cars. Inside, I checked in at 3:15 for a 3:30 p.m. appointment and took an uncomfortable seat outside the Imaging

Department. As the clock passed four and then five, I tried not to think about all I had to do. I tried not to think about how badly I wanted to be in India, how much I wanted my life to be different from how it was, and how uncomfortable and ominous the hospital waiting room felt.

I focused on the *New York Times* crossword puzzle, blocking out the people with oxygen tanks, walkers and hacking coughs who were crowding in around me. I was actively not looking at the woman who was too large to fit between the armrests when another, slimmer woman appeared before me.

"Hi, I'm Kara, and I'll be doing your MRI today."

We shook hands and I followed her through double doors into the neon-lit belly of the building. She wore blue scrubs and had her hair pulled back into a sloppy bun. She ushered me into a tiny changing room with a stack of gym lockers on the wall. "Take off your bra but leave your sweater on, and change out of your jeans and into these scrubs. Take off your jewelry and anything metal. You can lock everything in one of these lockers. There's a restroom next door, and I'll meet you in the hall right out here."

I didn't say anything. She looked at the clipboard in her hand.

"Hmmm," she said, running her finger down the page. "Your doctor ordered the MRI with and without contrast. We don't normally do contrast and it's going to cost you a lot if you're paying out of pocket."

I figured she was a doctor because we were in a hospital and she was wearing scrubs. When she looked up from the clipboard, though, she seemed more like a harried cocktail waitress on a busy Friday night. She had a look that said, "Know what you're having, honey? Cuz I've got lots of people waiting on another beer."

I didn't know what to say. I didn't know what I was having, and

I certainly didn't know what I was paying, even though I had insurance. When I had called to schedule this appointment, I forgot to ask what it would cost, so I asked when I checked in at the front desk. "With your insurance, you'll pay thirty percent," the receptionist said. "Thirty percent of what?" I asked.

She didn't know. She told me I could call financial services but that they wouldn't know either. "Maybe you could call tomorrow," she said, and directed me to the waiting room.

A couple of hours later and Kara was telling me this was going to cost a lot.

"What does that mean?" I asked, "How much?" as if price were my primary concern.

Kara said it depended on the number of cc's of the dye, which she called by name, as if that meant something to me. (I've since learned it's called gadolinium, and I still have no idea what it cost.) I didn't know the potential side effects and didn't think to ask, and she didn't mention them. The neurologist who ordered the MRI hadn't mentioned them either. All he said was that I should do this test sooner rather than later.

"I don't know," Kara said. "If you're paying out of pocket, could be five hundred dollars, maybe more."

This didn't seem like something a doctor would say—"could be five hundred dollars" seemed so imprecise—but I didn't have much experience with doctors.

"It's really unusual," she said. "Unless they're looking for something specific, we don't do it with and without contrast."

I stared at her. The room was so small and we were standing so close that I could see individual pores on her nose. I stared some more. "Look," I finally said. "My doctor must have ordered it for a reason," as if the neurologist were somebody I trusted or even knew well. After the fifteen minutes he spent with me, he was no more "my" doctor than she was.

"Here's what we'll do," Kara said, softening slightly. "We'll do it without contrast and if we can't get a clear picture, we'll do the contrast."

"I'm not coming back," I said, thinking, *I'm in India on Friday, I don't have time for this.*

She said a radiologist could look at the images while I was on the table, and we could add the contrast then, if necessary. Fine, done. She left the changing room. I took off my pants, stepped into the enormous scrubs, and took off my sweater. I was wearing a bra with stars on it. Wonder Woman.

I put my sweater back on, locked my stuff in a box, stepped into the hall and sat down on another uncomfortable chair that somewhere some factory snapped together by the thousands. I picked up an old copy of a personal finance magazine and flipped the pages while I cursed myself for all the missteps I must have made rushing headlong into this moment.

✚ ✚ ✚

The tingling had started six months earlier. It wasn't painful, just an annoying pins-and-needles in my fingertips. And on the list of things that needed attention in my life, the tingling wasn't alone. I'd gotten a divorce a year earlier and changed careers the year before that. In the aftermath, my life felt chaotic and confusing. I wanted to slow down, to take time to think and to find answers, so I planned a monthlong sabbatical to begin January 1. And while I was planning the trip to sort out big-picture questions, I tried to get rid of the tingling—which seemed small and unrelated. I saw a chiropractor and a physical therapist. Neither helped. After a while, I figured I should see a physician. At the time, I didn't have one, because I'd never needed one. And I had the cheapest insurance for the same reason: I'd been healthy my whole life.

The tingling, however, was persistent, so I selected a primary care physician off of my HMO's website. I picked her because she had curly hair like me. And I liked her name, Dr. Wise.

I made an appointment in late November and went to see her. When I explained the tingling, she poked my toes with a two-pronged, forklike thing, asking me to identify one or two prongs without looking. All my toes could count so she shrugged her shoulders and suggested a neurologist. She gave me a name and I booked an appointment.

In mid-December, I waited in his office, shivering in a paper gown for half an hour before a med student came in and did preliminary tests. The med student, a boyish-looking redhead, was basically the warm-up act, sent to entertain me and to practice his routine. He left and eventually returned with a gray-haired man who did the same tests. The older man said his name was Dr. Silver, and he asked me to follow his finger with my eyes. He hit my knees with a reflex hammer and watched as I did a few of the actual drunk-driving tests: *Shut your eyes, put your arms out straight then touch your nose with each first finger. Walk heel to toe, then stand on one foot and look at the sky.*

I could manage all of them, so Silver asked me to walk heel to toe backward. On this, my balance was embarrassingly bad. I'd pulled something in my hip a month earlier and tried to run on it anyway. When that didn't work, I stopped running for a while to let it rest and have time to heal without seeing a doctor. And by the time I met Silver, the pain was gone, but heel-to-toe walking backward was not in my repertoire. I explained this. He nodded.

After fifteen minutes, the quiet doctor had seen enough and suggested I get some blood tests and an MRI.

"I'm going to Seattle tomorrow, then I'm home for two days, and off to India for a month," I said. "Do I need to do this before I go?"

He said I should.

No stranger to last-minute changes, I spent Christmas with my cousins, cut the trip short and caught a flight home at six in the morning. I landed in Denver and found myself driving to one of the hospitals affiliated with my HMO. I gave what the phlebotomist assured me was no more than five tablespoons of blood for five different tests.

I ran a few errands and drove to another hospital for the 3:30 p.m. appointment. It was still one more item on my to-do list: pick up insect repellent, buy sunscreen, get an MRI, stop the mail.

After a two-hour wait in the main holding tank, and a quick and uncomfortable conversation with Kara, I was waiting again, this time in the hall outside the MRI room.

And for the first time since the tingling began, I had to acknowledge what I was feeling: fear.

Earlier in the day, I was in charge. Sure, my career was off track and my social life was "confused," but it was *my* life. I was sure of that, and I knew I wasn't sick, just slightly off track. I was going to India to sort it out. And after that, I was going to get on with my future.

That confidence faded as I sat in the waiting room surrounded by sick people, and it vanished completely in the closet with Kara. And as I waited some more, my optimism gave way to something more sinister. At half past five, with no new information, I became certain that I had something awful, irreversible, painful and hard to pronounce. And, as my brain was taking stock of this new situation, this "uh oh, I'm sick" situation, my body had the urge to bolt. I looked around and contemplated grabbing my stuff and sprinting back down the hallway, through the double doors, past the waiting room and out the main door into the cold, dry Colorado night. I saw myself running and holding the enormous blue scrubs at my waist so I didn't run right out of them.

Before I could make a move, though, Kara reappeared. She brought me into the darkened room and gave me a bolster to rest my knees and a warm blanket to cover me from toes to chest. Sliding into the tube was a little uncomfortable because it was close, but it wasn't unbearable. I shut my eyes and concentrated on my breathing.

The pounding started, and I told myself it didn't bother me. The MRI machine makes a *duh-duh-duh-duh-duh* sound like a jackhammer, which is annoying and not unfamiliar. I lived in New York City in the 1990s. Pounding, hammering, sirens—I made a habit of ignoring them all.

Two minutes of hammering was followed by twenty or thirty seconds of nothing, followed by another minute or two of hammering, and on and on. I focused on my breath and told myself this was no scarier than the dentist's office. And it wasn't, until Kara came back into the room.

"All right, we're not getting a clear picture of your spine so we have to do the contrast," she said, as I was sliding out of the MRI tube. She took my hand off my chest, unbent my elbow and started rubbing alcohol on my arm.

"That doesn't sound good," I said. "What do you mean, it's not a clear picture?" I thought she was telling me she was incompetent, that she hadn't focused the lens like an amateur photographer might miss a shot with a new camera.

"We can't get a clear image. There's plaque on your spinal cord. Spots that show up. It could be you. It could be MS. I don't know.

I'm not going to diagnose this right now," she said in a rapid stream of words and sounds.

*Wait, did she just say, "It could be MS?"*

I didn't know much about multiple sclerosis. Didn't matter. When Kara said, "It could be MS," my mind ran ahead to fill in all the blanks and gaps in what I did know. It sprinted past words to images of wheelchairs and dependency and pain.

"Spots that show up. It could be you. It could be MS. I don't know."

Remembering it now, I think I was supposed to feel my heart race or launch up into my head, accompanied by a panic shot of adrenaline. That's not what I felt.

I felt my heart drop down, falling through my back, through the table I was lying on, through the floor and into the earth. I felt my heart falling through dark and quiet earth, toward what I didn't know.

While my heart went on tour, my brain slowed down enough to take stock of the situation. "Are you a doctor?"

"No," she said. "I wish."

"Me too. Are you a nurse?"

"No," Kara said, and launched into a long story about how she'd been doing this for eighteen years and all the classes she had to take to keep her licensing current.

While she rambled on, I checked out of her monologue, stopped listening and started to panic again, until I zoned out completely.

Kara injected dye into my arm and I noticed a slight electric smell, like the air before lightning strikes, or maybe a taste. Suddenly, I was sliding back into the MRI machine. I concentrated on my breath and the knocking began again.

✚ ✚ ✚

I woke the next day still planning to go to India. The whole Kara incident had been relegated to the place in my mind where I leave bad dreams. I discounted what she said because she was merely a technician and not "my" doctor. And multiple sclerosis didn't sound right. I ran marathons, galloped horses, kayaked wonderfully cold water. I couldn't have MS. I knew there was another explanation, so I called Dr. Silver's office and asked if I could see him that day or the next.

The nurse, sweet as can be, chuckled. "Oh gosh, no, he's booked."

I explained that I'd just had a mess of blood tests and an MRI, and I was about to leave the country. "How can I get the results?"

She said she'd call me with the blood tests and let Dr. Silver know I wanted to hear from him.

"MRI readings," she said, "take time. The radiologist has to look at the images, write a report and find someone to dictate it so Dr. Silver can call and listen."

Only at the end of this elaborate game of telephone could Dr. Silver call me to tell me the results. Or I could check online while I was in India.

Check online? I was surprised and thrilled. No one would deliver bad news online. And since the nurse was being so nice, I thought she might offer sympathy for my rotten experience in the hospital. I told her about Kara the med tech diagnosing me with MS, and the nurse gasped.

"I don't know exactly how that hospital works, but call the main number and ask for the patient advocate and tell them the story. That's outrageous."

I hung up and looked at the card Kara had given me. It listed phone numbers for the hospital and the director of imaging. Kara had signed in a big loopy hand with a "Thanks!" and a smiley face.

Goddamn cocktail waitress.

I dialed the department director's line and left a detailed message. Then, I grabbed my bag and left to get that bug spray I still needed for India.

I was home at noon and beginning to clean my house when Silver called. He said he'd heard I had a rough experience at the imaging center and asked if I could tell him about it. "I'd like to know because I refer people there," he said.

I told him the story. He apologized and moved on. "There are lesions on your spinal cord and the most likely cause is MS."

"What? Really? I did not expect you to say that." I dropped the vacuum I was holding and fell back onto the couch. Then I stared at the ceiling unsure what else to say.

Silver jumped in. "If you want to talk about it, I can stay a little past my last patient today at four thirty."

"Um, yes, I do," I said. "I'll be there at four thirty."

I hung up and called a friend. She wasn't home, so I left a message. Then I started vacuuming the couch as if nothing had changed.

Within ten minutes, the tingling had spread from my fingers to my entire body. Every bit of me was screaming and shaking and demanding attention. I couldn't stand up. I couldn't sit down. I could hardly do anything other than panic.

I called my friend Jonathan, who is a life coach. Crying, I told him what Silver said. Jonathan had one word: *breathe*.

I told him I couldn't and that every part of my body was more than tingling. That it felt like an electrical storm running through my entire body.

"Right," he said, as if he'd seen this before. "Ten billion cells are wondering who's in charge over there. You have got to breathe. Breathe, in and out."

Jonathan listened as I inhaled and exhaled, uncomfortably at first.

When I settled into an easier rhythm, he said, "Think about your dog. You know how you can direct her to do something?"

Riley, my Australian shepherd, was already at the friend's who would watch her while I was in India. I pictured her tilting her head when I asked her to come, and I pictured the politician who had come to the door. The poor guy asked for my vote, and Riley sprung on to the porch and peed on his shoe.

"I guess she listens, maybe, sometimes," I said. "When it suits her."

"Jody," Jonathan said. "Use your mind to calm your body. Tell your body to relax. Tell your body you're in charge and that this is going to be OK. And breathe."

I did. Jonathan stayed on the phone for a while, and when we hung up, I sunk back into the couch and stared into space one more time.

I wanted someone bigger than me and stronger than me to tell me this would be OK. I wanted somebody to hold me together and tell me I was OK. I could think of only one person who could say anything in a way I might believe. His name was Bruce, and I'd met him too soon after my divorce to start dating and too soon after his. Yet, we had started. A Canadian with homes in Vancouver, London and Cabo San Lucas, Bruce was a charismatic businessman with a belief in Buddhist teachings.

I knew he was in Mexico and didn't always answer his phone when he was there. I sent an email saying, "My neurologist wants to see me at four thirty. This can't be good," and then I continued cleaning the house.

At four o'clock, my friend Rebecca arrived. I didn't want to go to Dr. Silver's alone. I thought I might be overwhelmed and wouldn't be able to take in all that the doc said. I thought I might not be able to drive.

I got in her car and we drove across town to the hospital. *Her car is really clean,* I thought. *It must be easier when you don't have a dog.*

At Silver's office, we waited a minute or twelve or twenty—it's hard to say—in the empty waiting room. Last time I was there I had made the mistake of reading *Neurology Today*, which is filled with stories of horrible neurological diseases and the people who live with them. I mentioned that and Rebecca said, "We won't do that again."

A nurse appeared and escorted us into Silver's office. She took my blood pressure and asked if I wanted anything. I couldn't think of anything. We waited some more.

Dr. Silver arrived and took a seat in the small room, now crowded with three of us and an examination table.

I have my notes. I have Rebecca's notes.

Mine are written the way I'd taken notes on any number of press conferences over the years. Or more accurately, the writing—the actual handwriting—is the same. Normally sports press conferences start with the coach or the athlete clearing his throat. "This is a great opportunity for our team to regroup," "I'm looking forward to the upcoming season," or "I'm resigning to spend more time with my family." In sports press conferences, people lead with the banal. The first page of notes could usually be tossed with no loss to the story being told.

Not here. In my notes from December 30, the second line reads: my own immune system attacking myself.

Rebecca's notes are remarkably thorough. She wrote down my blood pressure, 124 over 78, and a haiku-like version of everything Silver said:

*Blood brain barrier*
*Unique to nervous system*
*Doesn't go into brain*

And

*Diabetes, say,*
*Would be shown in blood tests*
*That's not what this is*

And then there's a line similar to the one I wrote. And it's just as hideous in either hand: "immune system tries to attack own nervous system—multiple sclerosis."

At the time, all I could think was, *What the hell? That makes no sense*. Even now, when I read it, that's what I think. *Really? The immune system attacks the nervous system? Like they don't know they're on the same team? That's fucked up.*

Usually with MS, Silver explained, a person has gotten a virus as a child, and the immune system kicked in and did what it's supposed to do. It creates lymphocytes that attack the virus. When they've done their job, and the virus is dead and gone, the lymphocytes go dormant. Then, for some reason, in some people, something triggers those same lymphocytes to spring back into action decades later. They go to work again, only they have no virus to attack. Instead, they attack the central nervous system.

"We don't know why," he said.

As frustrating as his theory was, I had no other thoughts or explanations. I hadn't done any research, because until that moment, MS didn't affect me as far as I knew. And the return of some dormant attack cells was the story the doctor was telling, so who was I to question him? He was the authority in the room, calling me Jody while I called him Doctor. He wore the white coat, rattled off medical speak and sat before a collection of framed diplomas on the wall. I sat trembling on a small stool with a note pad on my lap.

"The most common primary diagnosis in young women is MS," Silver said. "Perhaps it's tied to women's genetic makeup."

"I'm not that young," I said.

"You're young enough."

He added that most often MS is a series of active disease episodes, or "flare-ups," followed by periods of remission. What happens early, he said, doesn't predict how the disease goes later. Then he moved to discussing treatment.

Silver was already calling the tingling in my hands "a flare-up," as though there were no question the cause was MS. The way to treat it, he said, was with a short pulse of steroids to suppress the immune system.

"I can't suppress my immune system and go to a third-world country."

"Well, it's not ideal, but I'm a doctor and we work to keep people going in their lives. This trip is part of your life. Let's talk about it, about where you're going and what the risk factors are."

I was flying into Chennai, a city of five million people in the southern Indian state of Tamil Nadu. I was to spend a few days there, tour a few temples and drive to the coast for ten days at the Quiet Healing Center for a yoga retreat.

"Again, it's not my first choice, but you're not going to be in any of the big cities so the risk is lower," Silver said. I didn't question whether a city of five million counted as big before he launched into possible side effects of the high dose of steroids. Upset stomach, anxiety, bloating, sleeplessness and others.

He said doctors used to prescribe long doses of steroids for MS, but now they hit it hard for a short time and a quick taper. He talked about 1,000 milligrams a day for four days. Although, he said, statistically that's more likely to cause the side effects.

Because I was about to catch a plane, he prescribed 500 milligrams a day for four days and a longer taper. Then he went through the side effects again. When he got to the sleeplessness part, he flipped to a new page on his pad and, without looking up, started scribbling. "I can prescribe a sleeping pill," he said.

The sleeping pill scared me more than the steroids did. "Hang on," I said. "I don't even take aspirin."

I had stopped taking over-the-counter medications ten years earlier. One spring the pollen counts reached record highs and my nose ran constantly, my eyes watered and my throat itched. I tried several allergy pills and felt like I was auditioning for the Seven Dwarfs. I went from Sneezy to Sleepy, to Dopey, to Grouchy—or is it Grumpy? Years before that, nighttime cold medications kept me awake for three days, and something that promised to settle my stomach left me so disinterested in food that I skipped five meals. Finally, with the allergy meds, I realized that over-the-counter drugs were not engineered for me. I never tried them again.

My mistrust was even more pronounced with sleeping pills. When I lived in New York, everyone I knew took Ambien or some variation to fall asleep at night. And that's one of the reasons I left. I didn't want to live in a city where medication was mandatory. I didn't think I could. And back in my arrogant thirty-third year, sleeping pills proved that life was out of balance—for others, those folks who took Ambien. Now, ten years later, it seemed my life was the one that was hopelessly and irretrievably out of balance.

Silver didn't seem to hear me. "Really," I repeated. "I don't take aspirin."

"Neither do I," he said, and I believed him. He said it almost apologetically, and he looked the type to eat well, abstain from drugs and alcohol, and run a tidy five miles every morning or play squash with his old boarding-school buddies.

"Statistically," he said, "most people have no reaction. If you were going to have one, it would happen in the first forty-eight hours. It's tight but," he looked at his watch, "go to the pharmacy now and we have almost forty-eight hours until you board the flight."

Rebecca and I looked at the clock: five thirty. The pharmacy closed at six. My flight left Denver International Airport forty-one hours later, at 10:30 a.m. on January 1.

Silver wrote three prescriptions: one for Ambien and two for Prednisone. I still have the Ambien.

Rebecca had one more question: "So, is there anything she shouldn't do?"

"I wouldn't do crystal meth," Silver said so evenly that a moment passed before we registered the joke.

Rebecca forged ahead: "It's New Year's tomorrow. Can she have a drink?"

Silver said sure, everything in moderation.

Right.

CHAPTER 2

# SOLO AT DUO

Rebecca and I left Dr. Silver's office and rode the elevator in silence. We walked to the pharmacy and waited while the woman behind the counter counted little pills into three little bottles. She asked if I understood the directions on how to take them. I nodded and she gave me directions anyway, in an impersonal prerecorded tone.

"Do you want to get something to eat?" Rebecca asked as we walked to the car. "What's comfort food for you?"

"There's a great restaurant in my neighborhood, Duo. Do you know it?"

As we drove, I could barely think about what just happened. It was as if the stress was so great that my brain had just refused to consider the conversation with Silver or its implications. And my mind simply refused to acknowledge my fear. All I could think of was food. And I wasn't that hungry.

No, I craved comfort, and Duo's roast chicken with smashed sweet potatoes and some kind of warm, wilted greens is as comforting as anything I could imagine. And more than the food, the place was calming. Softly lit and warm with the smells of freshly baked bread, the feel was the opposite of the hospital with its neon lights and harsh voices.

We took a table between the bar and the kitchen, which is open for all to see. And I wanted to see. I cooked in restaurants through college and still enjoyed the sounds of kitchen chatter. Missed being a part of it, really. And for a few minutes at Duo, I could be a part of it. I could imagine myself standing with those men in white jackets behind the line. I could feel the satisfaction of teamwork, the knowledge that three people created three totally different dishes that appeared steaming hot all at the same time. And I knew the game of giving a waitress grief for not being there at the precise moment of triumph.

As I watched the cooks, I pictured my line, the guys I cooked with. Me, Mark and Mark—we were like one of the great lines in hockey, moving as one organism, dishing, delivering and cracking each other up. We didn't work in an open kitchen, so occasionally, when things were slow, we'd try juggling. All kinds of round things sit in a kitchen so we'd grab a tomato, a grapefruit and an egg—or some other unlikely combination. I didn't know how to juggle, and only one of the Marks almost did. We giggled like schoolgirls as each of us tried to keep three objects in the air and then pass them to one another. It didn't matter where raw egg splattered. We were having a ball and we could try again the next day.

While I was sitting and staring toward one kitchen in Denver, imagining another kitchen at another time in Durham, North Carolina, a tall waitress came to our table. I asked for the roast chicken and a glass of wine. Rebecca told the waitress that she was vegan and that what she really wanted was one side dish from one entrée and another from a different entrée. "Would that be OK?"

The waitress said of course, collected our menus and walked

away. I felt like I was watching a movie. Like I wasn't really the one sitting there having just been diagnosed with something awful. Like I wasn't alone but felt for the girl on the screen who was. Like I was still the girl cooking my way through college, knowing that I could do anything I wanted, once I knew what I wanted.

The food arrived and as we ate, Rebecca talked about her doctor and how she had a great doctor but most people didn't. "I'm really lucky," she said. "I have a great doctor—really, really great. And a great dentist too. I'm really lucky I found them. And I have a great massage therapist too. She's amazing, can heal anything. She's really good with MS."

Rebecca chattered about Kathie, the massage therapist, and how long Rebecca had been going to her and how she cured her anxiety and really helped her with anything going on in her body. "I'm so lucky I found all of them," Rebecca said. "Most people just don't have the kind of support that I do."

I stared at her.

She kept talking and I kept staring. I wasn't the only one feeling the stress from Silver's office. And maybe most people, hearing that a friend was diagnosed with something awful, would think, "I'm glad it's not me."

I wondered how many people would come so close to saying it out loud.

When our food arrived, I took a slow sip of the wine. It tasted summery compared to the chill outside and the hearty roasted chicken and root vegetables on my plate. I looked at Rebecca, watched her mouth making words, and wondered how I could be sitting in Duo, knowing that I was completely and unquestionably solo: *How come I am so alone? How did I set up my life so that when I desperately need someone to care for me, to tell me it's going to be OK, I've got no one? What was I thinking?*

And as my mind moved to answer that question, I had to inhale sharply to cut off an explosion of tears: *I can't have MS. This won't work. People with MS need people to take care of them. And I've got no one. I can't have MS.*

I couldn't stay with that thought; it was too scary. I looked around the room, looked back at Rebecca and took another sip of wine.

We finished dinner, and while we waited for the check, I took a handful of Prednisone out of the little yellow bottle. Five tiny white pills, each the size of a pinhead. I counted them a couple of times, swallowed them and took another sip of wine. And then some water. Water seemed like a good idea.

When the check came, Rebecca said, "I'm just going to put in five dollars because all I had was vegetables. And water. I didn't have anything to drink."

"Oh," I said, a little confused and mostly numb. I stared at the bill and then at her and said, "Oh, OK. That's fine."

Bruce called when we were in the car. "Can I call you back in a sec when I'm in my house?"

"Sure," he said, "no problem. But call me back."

Rebecca dropped me off, and when I got inside, my house felt odd, like there was a sheet of glass between me and everything around me. It was cold, and like all of Colorado in the winter, the air was perfectly dry and still. For the second time that night, I felt like I was on a movie set, like no one really lived there.

I made a cup of tea and sunk into the big couch to dial Bruce.

We'd known each other a little over a year, and although we hadn't lived in the same place or spent more than a week at a time together, he was the one I wanted to talk to. He was the only one. Bruce was big and strong, physically and emotionally, and I knew I needed that.

"Hey, sweetie, what's going on?"

I told him that there were lesions on my spinal cord. I couldn't say MS. If I said it to him, or out loud to anyone, I'd be acquiescing. I'd be saying that, yes, my immune system was attacking my central nervous system. Even though I was terrified that this was true, and even though I'd left Silver's office, went to the pharmacy and dutifully swallowed a fistful of Prednisone, I wasn't so sure.

Bruce asked the obvious question, "What does that mean?"

"I don't know."

Silver thought he knew, and in a state of panic, I was following his directions. Still, I had my doubts. I didn't *really* know what the lesions meant. After all, Silver had spent fifteen minutes with me before ordering the MRI and declaring the diagnosis. Fifteen minutes didn't seem like enough to make such a serious and permanent pronouncement. *My immune system attacking my central nervous system? Really?* To Silver, that didn't seem outlandish. Maybe he believed that it was the only explanation for the tingling in my fingers. Or maybe his faith in his education and experience made asking questions or listening to answers irrelevant. Maybe medical school, an MRI and his instincts told him all he needed to know.

I needed more.

I believe interviews are valuable and that good ones take time. I have interviewed thousands of athletes, coaches, trainers and fans over a dozen years as a sportswriter. No one, to my knowledge, ever gave up anything good in the first fifteen minutes. Generally, at that point, the subject was still coming to terms with the idea of an interview, still sorting out, consciously or subconsciously, what the questioner was seeking and deciding whether to help or hinder the search.

"What are lesions?" Bruce asked.

"I think they're like bruises. He showed me the MRI. He flashed it on a computer screen and he pointed to stuff but I don't know.

It's like the first time you go to a planetarium and some guy's saying this is Orion's Belt and the sword of something or other, and all you see are stars."

I didn't want to repeat Silver's explanation of the image on his screen. I was afraid to tell anyone—especially someone I loved—that I might be sick. I grew up thinking illness and injury were shameful acts. My Grandma Ann lived nearby, and I met her only once, by accident. I knew three grandparents well—had dinner with them weekly and saw them for holidays. But my dad's mom, long divorced from his dad, was only a name until one day she rang the doorbell. I was in third grade. I had just gotten home from school, and I don't know where my sister was. My mom answered the door and let my grandma in but told her she couldn't stay, that she had to leave before my dad came home. I don't think Grandma Ann was offered a seat. She came into the kitchen, gave my mom a small Torah scroll, said hello to me and left.

When she was gone, my mom told me not to tell my dad. I asked why, and my mom said that Grandma Ann was a sick woman.

Years later, my mom would tell me that Grandma Ann had schizophrenia. And that was all. I never learned about her symptoms, who diagnosed her or what the treatment was. I was only told that she was sick. And at eight years old, all I knew was that she was sick and we didn't know her. She wasn't welcome in our house.

"How are you feeling?" Bruce asked.

"I don't know. A little spacey right now."

I was afraid that if I told him what Silver said, I would be abandoned, locked out of the house. And with Bruce, I was afraid it might be tough for him too.

His ex-wife had just died. Although they had divorced before she passed away (and well before I met him), they had remained close, and he always looked out for her. He was there for her as skin cancer spread through her liver, lungs and brain. For two years, he was on the phone or sitting with her as she struggled and suffered through all kinds of experimental treatments. Bruce let his hopes ride and fall with hers each time, with each treatment, and always paid the bill. In her last months, as she came in and out of a coma, Bruce sat with her reading from the *bardos* in the *Tibetan Book of the Dead*. He read to her every day until she closed her eyes and let go.

She had let go in late October. And now, here we were in December. And I was telling him (or avoiding telling him) that I might be sick too.

Bruce listened to me even though I was talking without saying much. I mumbled around and he listened. He sounded concerned and confused—as I was. Eventually, I remembered that this was Bruce on the other end of the line; that he was solid and knew how to be there for someone in sickness; and that I could tell him anything, that I always told him everything, even when the words coming out of my mouth surprised me.

I remembered that I loved him. I tentatively trotted out the *M* word.

"There are experts in that field in Vancouver," he said. "We will get you in to see them. I don't think you have it. And whatever it is, we'll take care of it."

I believed him. Mentally and physically, I believed him. After an entire day of unconsciously clenching my shoulders up near my ears, I felt them relinquish their perch and slide down my back to where they belonged.

I exhaled and heard Bruce do the same.

"You're not going to India tomorrow, are you, babe? It's the next day, right? Get a good night's sleep and call me in the morning."

We hung up and I looked around the room. The heavy sectional couch that I should not have taken in the divorce was too big for the room, and the framed photo too small on the far wall. I thought about going to sleep, although it wasn't a serious option. Internally, I was firing at full speed. I could feel my body aching to move, to go somewhere, to do something. I walked into the kitchen as if an urgent task awaited me there, and then realized I could Google "MS." And as soon as I remembered that Google existed, I felt like an idiot that I hadn't thought of it before. I had been a reporter—nationally recognized, award winning—and a lot of good it did me in that moment. Writing for newspapers and magazines, I had been dedicated to research and did copious amounts before any event. If I had to cover a Little League game, I would have called the coach, chatted with him and asked for the name of a parent to call. Then I would have dialed the parent, chatted with her and asked for more people to talk to. I might have made six calls and studied stats before going to a baseball game that even the players would soon forget.

I had built a career like that, digging into, exploring and explaining other people's lives. I would have gone to a Little League game with more information and having asked more questions and collected more context than I had or did before going to the hospital to see Dr. Silver. In prepping to learn about my own body, I hadn't even done the simplest thing—a Google search.

I went into my office and sat down at the big oak desk, a solid piece of furniture that had once lived in the old Denver Public Library. I fired up my tiny laptop and went to the almost-unavoidable search engine.

Just type in a question and Google shoots out an answer: it's almost a public service. Yet in moments of rapid-fire insecurity, that beast is dangerous friend.

The National MS Society website said MS isn't an easy disease to diagnose, that there's no single test for it, and that the diagnosis cannot be made until the doctor finds evidence of two episodes of disease activity in the central nervous system that have occurred at different points in time.

*Wait, two?! I didn't have two episodes, just one long tingling. Why was it so easy for Silver to diagnose, then?*

The Mayo Clinic's website said that multiple sclerosis is a potentially debilitating disease in which your body's immune system eats away at the protective sheath that covers your nerves. Great. I must need that sheath; it must be important for something. Why would my body attack it? Why would my own body attack me?

I searched the Centers for Disease Control. There I learned that MS is a progressive and usually fluctuating disease with exacerbations and remissions over many decades. In many patients with MS, according to the CDC, permanent disability and even death can occur. Awesome. *How can I travel around the world to sit in hero's pose when I might be dying?*

I kept searching, and the more I searched, the less I knew. The more I read, the scarier everything became. MS seemed completely inscrutable and could include any number of symptoms: it could mean paralysis or pain or vision problems. It could include weakness, incontinence and a number of other things. The ambiguity terrified me.

As I considered this, the phone rang. I was hoping it was Bruce calling back, but it was Joan, a friend of my friend Jonathan. I'd forgotten he had asked if a friend could call. At the time, I didn't think to ask who she was, why she would call, or why I would want to talk to her.

And now here she was. Joan introduced herself, in a sweet soft voice, and said she'd heard about my day. I walked back to the living room and sank back into the couch as she launched into her story of being diagnosed with MS when she was twenty-three years old. She was running a division of an advertising agency, playing semi-pro beach volleyball and training for a triathlon when her feet went numb. No big deal, she thought, and assumed she'd taken a bad fall on the volleyball court.

A month later she had no feeling in either leg. She went to a doctor who wanted to admit her for tests. She had no time and left. And a month after that, Joan returned in a wheelchair. She had lost the use of both legs. That was twenty-three years earlier.

I sat curled on the couch, wrapped in a blanket and wishing my dog were home to comfort me. Because I was exhausted or stunned or stupid (or some combination of all three, enhanced by steroids), I once again acted as if I'd never been a reporter. I failed to ask a single question as Joan detailed her horrifying descent into hell.

My brain was racing along and I couldn't slow it down long enough to pick anything apart. There seemed to be no opening for me to say, even to myself, "Hold on, why am I listening to this woman I don't know? Is any of this true? And does it matter to me?"

Joan kept talking. She was a good storyteller. She'd told this story before, knew when to pause for effect, knew how to *sell* it.

"In the beginning," Joan said, "I did everything the doctors told me to do." She told me about the interferon drugs prescribed to alter the course of the disease and how she injected herself on schedule. Even though the sight of her injection sites would clear out the pool, she continued to swim when she could. "Swimming is really good for MS patients," she said, as if we were in some club together.

She said she'd had annual and awful "flare-ups," which included bouts of blindness and paralysis until eleven years in, she drove her car into a head-on collision that proved a wake-up call.

In the hospital as she recovered, Joan wondered about taking the drugs and all the suffering. She began to think the two might be related. She told me she had stopped taking her medications and had been symptom-free ever since.

Symptom-free! I didn't know this woman—couldn't pick her out of a police lineup—and before she called I didn't even know I was afraid of going blind suddenly or losing the use of my legs. Now, in no time at all, I went from being panicked, numb and too terrified to speak to being fully and completely relieved. As in, extraordinary, jumping-for-joy, "I could kiss this woman and scream out loud" relieved.

I was ecstatic. I didn't have to go blind. Didn't have to end up in a wheelchair. Didn't even have to take the drugs. Joan had figured out how to avoid all that. I could too.

Her optimism was a world away from the doomsday pamphlets Silver had given me and my gloomy Google search. Joan credited her remarkable recovery to two things—a strict and extensive vitamin regimen and time spent at Sanoviv, a holistic healing center in Mexico. She talked about the extensive assessments they do there, testing for nutritional deficiencies, heavy metal toxicities, physical strength and flexibility. She lavished praise on the wonderfully team-based approach to healing.

As Joan talked about doctors and medications and vitamins and theories, she spoke fast, without breathing, as if this were critical information she was imparting. And with Prednisone sluicing through my veins, I felt like I'd downed a few espressos and was waiting for a few more. Joan could have cranked the RPMs higher still and I would have been right with her.

Joan told me about Dr. Paolo Zamboni, an Italian researcher who had discovered a correlation with MS and blocked veins in the neck.

He devised an angioplasty-like treatment. "It's called CCSVI and it's the talk of the MS world," Joan said.

Before I could ask why she was still researching experimental options in Italy if she'd found the answer in Mexico, she asked about India.

"What are you planning to do there?" Joan asked.

"Practice yoga and meditate."

"Couldn't you do that in Colorado?"

The answer of course was yes.

"The time in India isn't what I'd worry about," Joan said. "It's all the time in airports, standing and waiting in line, and sitting on those long flights."

I didn't disagree. As a journalist, I had traveled all over the world. I had covered surfing in Fiji, adventure racing in Ecuador, diving in the Cayman Islands and the Olympics on three continents. For a dozen years, I flew once a week, sometimes more, and spent more time in airports and hotels than is healthy for anybody. I loved airplanes, taking off and landing in a new place. Airports, however, with their illogical lines and lousy food, had always unsettled me. And now, with a suppressed immune system and untold side effects from the Prednisone looming in my immediate future, airports and even airplanes seemed terrifying.

As if Joan and I were old friends, or even family, we discussed the ups and downs of going to India—mostly the downs: standing in the security line, inhaling other people's coughs and sneezes, and sitting on two ten-hour flights, breathing only recycled air. After all that, India no longer seemed a safe spot to land.

I wanted to go. I needed to go. I had planned for it and finally had time to go. Yet now, all of a sudden, another quest was taking over. I needed to know what was going on in my body. And Joan had a point too: Could I enjoy India while my mind galloped away on a steroid-sponsored hamster wheel? Could I even try to meditate when my mind seemed to be everywhere except in my body and in this moment? What if my life was going to include sudden bouts of blindness?

Crap.

When I hung up, I didn't know what to do. Maybe my life would be like Joan said hers was now: I'd get off the Prednisone and take vitamins, the tingling would leave, and I'd be completely symptom-free. Or maybe my life would be like hers when she was first diagnosed, with weeks or months of unpredictable disabilities. I couldn't go to India not knowing which version the future held. I fell asleep "knowing" I would cancel my flight. I also knew if that felt wrong in the morning, I could make a different decision.

At two in the morning, I looked at the clock and wondered if I should go. At three thirty, I did it again. I stared at the ceiling for a while and checked the clock again. Four thirty. Each time, I'd say I wasn't going, just to see how it felt.

By sunrise, it felt right. I got out of bed, took a handful of Prednisone and plotted a course to undo my travel plans.

CHAPTER 3

# OH NO, NOT INDIA

I couldn't reach Mitra. She was already in India with no phone and no access to email. And she was the reason I was going. She *was* India for me and now I wasn't going and I couldn't tell her.

I had met Mitra five years earlier, when friends invited me on a yoga retreat in Mexico. I'd never been to Mexico, rarely practiced yoga and had never been on a retreat of any kind. I signed up anyway, flew from Denver to Zihuatanejo (a name I could barely pronounce) and drove thirty minutes north to Troncones, a spectacularly quiet town along a strip of stunning white sand and a surprisingly noisy ocean. The group was large: fifteen women, one man, one mother and daughter pair, and me. Mitra was our teacher.

"I'm so glad you're here," she said immediately. It felt sincere and sweet even though we'd just met. And I was the only newcomer. She'd been taking students to Mexico twice a year for several years, and the others were her regular students from Santa Cruz, California.

Still, she hugged me. All five feet two inches of her hugged me. And then she stood back, beaming, with her long, flowing sari and an armful of bangles, and smiling like a little kid.

The next morning, all of us women and the lone guy met a different Mitra, a teacher on task, at eight in the morning in the *palapa*, a thatched-roof, open-sided studio on the beach. She stood at the front and waited while we settled onto our mats. When we were quiet, she spoke a quick and solemn-sounding line of Sanskrit, which we earnestly repeated.

Mitra then launched into two hours of intense instruction, calling out poses by their Sanskrit names that would have been foreign to me in any language. *Bhujangasana* meant as much or as little to me as "cobra pose"—which is to say nothing at all. With each pose, I'd look around and try to copy what others were doing. Sometimes, I think I got close. Other times, Mitra would come over and adjust me, physically. As in, pick all of me up by my arms or by my ankles and completely realign me as if I were a Barbie doll. "Better?" she'd ask. I'd nod or smile.

While we stayed in place, sitting with each pose for minutes and minutes and *minutes*, Mitra talked philosophy. She told us what her teachers had told her—about the body, about the mind, about the universe. She talked about chakras and energy, breathing, and different Hindu deities.

Toward the end of the class, Mitra said something, and everyone around me kneeled and then sat down, between their feet. "*Suptavirasana*," Mitra said. *Huh?* I tried to follow.

"*Virasana* is hero's pose," Mitra said, "and *supta* means reclining."

Around me, the women and one man started leaning back onto their elbows. From there, they settled down further, laying on the floor with their knees still bent and a foot beside either hip. Their faces relaxed.

Still sitting upright, I studied them in amazement, and with agony in my feet.

"Here," Mitra said, handing me a block. "Sit on this and protect your knees. Don't lean back."

I placed the purple foam beneath my butt and felt better.

"If you keep practicing," Mitra said, "one fine day, your muscles will lengthen and relax, and you will sit easily into this hero's pose. One fine day."

*Yeah. One fine day.*

Class wound down, and we moved to the café for breakfast. Over eggs and avocados, we asked one another questions and listened the way you can when you have all the time in the world and no place else you need to be. When the plates were empty and the coffee long cold, people slowly drifted apart, moving to hammocks or walking on the beach or wading into the surf.

Late in the afternoon, we found one another again in the *palapa* and practiced for another two hours before eating dinner together as a group.

We did this every day—yoga in the morning, leisurely breakfast and fun on the beach, followed by more yoga and more food together. By the end of the week, all of us in this unlikely crew felt like we'd known one another always. And even "one fine day" felt familiar. Or at least the poses felt possible. Not this week, or even this year, but some day. If I continued to practice, I'd get there. One day, I would sit like a hero. I'd even recline and smile.

On the final morning, I hugged everyone and kissed Mitra goodbye. I promised her I'd come back. We both cried and hugged harder. I flew to Colorado, and she flew to California.

I didn't go back to Troncones for a long time, and I didn't stay in touch with Mitra, or with the others I met on that retreat. I had wanted to, had planned to, but didn't.

Back in Denver, other plans took over. Plans that sounded so normal. I got married. We bought a house. We furnished it and invited his parents to visit. And I worked, often and a lot. A recently retired journalist, I called myself a "communications consultant," but the title was more aspirational than actual. I went to awkward networking events and uncomfortable coffee meetings in search of clients. My husband was also struggling professionally, so I looked for work for him too. At night and on weekends, we drank expensive bottles of wine with other couples and never considered whether we were moving toward something we wanted.

Not surprisingly, we weren't.

My husband, who had been kind, quiet and just out of reach, grew angry and sullen. I matched his anger and added sadness. We tried counseling and gave up. He called a moving company one afternoon and booked a one-way flight back to his hometown of Sydney, Australia. I forced him to meet me at the courthouse to sign paperwork the day he was leaving.

And then he was gone and I had no one to cry with.

Three weeks later, I met Bruce and fell for his passion and power. He ran several companies, and when he wanted to see me, he'd move a board meeting to Colorado, forcing a dozen men to fly to Denver so he could work with them all day and have dinner with me at night. Or he'd fly me to France.

Clients also started showing up, so I had work to do. I didn't enjoy it, but it paid the bills, and I was flying to Nice on Friday. Or Mexico. Or someplace else to see Bruce.

When the tingling started, I had a sense that it was a sign. I thought it meant I wasn't taking care of myself.

The sensation started in June, ten months after my husband left and nine months after Bruce arrived, and it came and went all summer. One night, in late August, the tingling was enough to keep me awake. As I lay in bed, I tried to think about what would make it go away, what would feel like home.

Even though I hadn't seen Mitra in years, I thought of that trip to Troncones. I fell asleep thinking I needed to find her.

I didn't have to. One week later I received an email from her announcing a trip to India. She was taking students to practice yoga and tour the temples in her spiritual home. I had a few questions. And I knew that however Mitra answered, I was going to go. Some coincidences are impossible to ignore.

When I got her on the phone, she squealed. I told her I'd been planning to find her when the email arrived. "*Om namah shivaya*," she said. "I bow to the divine that resides within all of us."

"*Om namah shivaya.*"

We both giggled.

"You'll love it," Mitra said. "We're going to Auroville. It's the community Mother started. It's where she taught."

Mother, a spiritual teacher in southern India, was Mitra's North Star.

And talking to Mitra, I wanted to see what that felt like. I wanted a North Star. And I knew the trip to India was exactly what I needed—a little adventure in an exotic place and quiet, calm, contemplative time. Simply perfect.

That was in September. Now, in late December, after my time with Dr. Silver, I had to make other plans.

I couldn't call Mitra. Couldn't ask her advice, couldn't tell her what had happened, couldn't hear her voice. However, I could call—and really had to call—Lauren, who was going with me.

Lauren and I had been friends for a couple of years. She was ten years older and six inches shorter than me, and when other friends sided with my ex-husband in the divorce, she picked me. Or more accurately, Lauren and Pete, her husband of twenty-five years, didn't pick. They stayed friends with both of us. And at the time, when relationships seemed so fragile, that seemed a huge gift, a kindness I could never repay.

Lauren hadn't traveled much internationally. She had gotten her first passport only the year before and was ready to use it. Her husband didn't like to leave the county, let alone the country, so Lauren suggested that she and I travel together. I told her about India and forwarded Mitra's email to her.

Lauren read it and called right away. "Is it going to feel like a bunch of rich American women on a spa vacation?" she asked. "Is it going to feel like any spa anywhere? I want to feel like I've gone to another country."

When I relayed this to Mitra, she laughed. "When you cross the street, you have to look both ways to avoid monkeys and cows," she said. "You will feel like you are in India."

That seemed to satisfy Lauren, who somehow overcame her hesitation without asking the obvious questions. The week before we were to leave, she asked me, "Did you know that there's yoga every day?"

Yes, I knew. That's why I was going.

And then at the last minute I wasn't going. The day before the trip I called Lauren and told her. I didn't tell her the reason because it didn't feel safe. I had no idea what was going to happen next, and I wasn't ready to give away an incomplete story to let others fill in the blanks.

Not surprisingly, Lauren was unsatisfied. She begged me to tell her. She pressured me. She begged again.

"OK," I said finally. "But you've got to promise you won't tell anyone. I don't know what I think about this and I'm not ready to tell anyone."

"Of course I won't tell anyone, Jody. Just tell me."

I told her, and later I went to her house to drop off paperwork she needed for the trip. I sat with Lauren and her husband at their kitchen table. We made an odd threesome. Lauren is small and blond with wire-rimmed glasses. Pete, tall and dark with enormous hands and a full belly, is ten years her senior. And me, well, at that moment, it was hard to know who I was or explain how I got there.

"My brother has MS," Pete said.

"He was diagnosed seventeen years ago and probably had it before that," Lauren said. "He's fine. He gets around OK. He has a guy who lifts him out of bed in the morning."

My head emptied. Truly emptied like I'd been hit with a right cross to the temple.

I sat in silence.

Pete asked if Lauren would be OK in India without me, if Mitra would take care of her. "Of course," I said in a daze. "Of course. Mitra's an amazing woman. Lauren will have an unforgettable time."

I drove home in shock. *He's fine. He gets around OK. He has a guy who lifts him out of bed in the morning.*

Nothing about that sounded fine. Nothing.

And it felt dismissive, like, *What are you worried about? You'll just get some guy to pull you out of bed each day too.*

Aside from an initial flurry of emails from Lauren's friends writing to say they were sorry to hear I had MS and a voice mail from Pete, telling me not to worry, that Lauren was having a great time, I didn't hear from them after that. I'd never felt so alone in my life.

## CHAPTER 4

# RETURN TO SILVER

Without India, January was a black hole. No plans in Colorado. No calls coming in. I could devote myself full-time to untangling this mess. And as soon as I realized it would be a full-time job, I was exhausted by it and didn't want anything to do with it.

After precisely four days, I was done with MS. I didn't believe it. I didn't want it. And I didn't want Silver to believe I had it. I wanted him to tell me he'd made a mistake. I wanted him to apologize and give me back my old life, the one where I could fly to a foreign country without a worry in the world.

And if he wasn't going to realize and apologize for the error of his ways, I would do the reporting. I would dig in and find that proof, irrefutable proof, that he'd made a mistake. And of course he would concur and apologize.

Clearly, I didn't know doctors that well.

It didn't occur to me that I might not trust him. If I didn't trust him to say I was sick, then why would I believe him if he said I wasn't? I also didn't realize, not then, that I could get second and third and fourth opinions, or that my opinion was the one that mattered. With credibility sewn into his white coat and framed in diplomas on the wall, Silver seemed important. His opinion mattered. And I thought I could use the tools of my trade to sway that opinion.

I went to the back bedroom, my home office, to get to work. I looked out the window and wondered whether I should go to the grocery store or pick up my dog. I wondered whether my car needed an oil change and a half dozen other irrelevant things, all in an instant, before I remembered what I was doing at my desk. *Damn steroids*, I thought and went to the "Diagnosing Tools" page of the National MS Society website, which seemed to make it pretty clear that this disease was no match for fifteen minutes and an MRI:

> *Because there are no laboratory tests or particular symptoms that definitively point to a diagnosis of MS, confirming the diagnosis can be a complex process. It is not unusual for people to be told they have MS when they actually have something else, or for the diagnosis to be missed in people who actually have MS. Before confirming an MS diagnosis, the doctor must rule out any other condition that could be causing your symptoms.*

For a doctor to rule out MS, the site listed eight items, including Lyme disease, lupus, genetic disorders, structural damage to the spine and a vitamin B deficiency. I didn't want lupus or a genetic disorder, but a vitamin B deficiency sounded pretty good.

I Googled on. Over a variety of websites, I found convergence on the three requirements to diagnose: a doctor must identify multiple episodes, identify multiple lesions, and rule out everything else.

I believed that Silver had seen multiple lesions. I'm sure that's what he was trying to show me when he flashed the black-and-white image on his computer screen. Of the other two items, identifying multiple episodes and ruling out everything else, I felt shortchanged—as if I'd been sentenced without standing trial. I made an appointment to see Dr. Silver again and started writing down a list of questions.

On a yellow legal pad, I wrote down "hepatitis A," "polio booster" and "tetanus." Because of the India trip, I had just had shots for all three. Did that matter? What about heavy metal toxicity? Could that be the cause of this? I had seen a chiropractor who said my spine was out of alignment. Could that be what this is? The tingling gained volume after a stressful day at work and an aggressive session with the chiropractor. Doesn't that mean something?

I'd had digestive problems several months before the tingling started. And a weird rash months before that. The dermatologist I saw handed me preprinted pages off her prescription pad. Could the tingling be a reaction to the antibiotics and corticosteroids she gave me? *Note to self: Where was my "I don't take medication" story then?*

On January 4, I drove myself back to the hospital and realized I had knowledge I never wanted: I knew exactly where to park and where to check in. I was already writing a check for the fifty-dollar co-pay when the woman at reception called my file up on her screen. "Know how to get to Neurology?" she asked.

"Yep," I said, sadly.

I came armed with a book this time to avoid the hazards in the waiting room. But sitting in the uncomfortable and cold space, I read a handful of pages and couldn't tell what they were about. Cursing the Prednisone, as was becoming my habit, I started to reread the same pages when a nurse stuck her head into the waiting area.

"Ms. Berger?"

She had strawberry-blond hair and a roundish face. I followed her down the hall and into an examining room. Even though I had come armed this time, fully prepared with my book, a list of questions and a sturdy disbelief in the diagnosis, my resolve diminished as soon as we stepped into the harshly lit room. I looked at the metal examining table, the tiny metal sink and the antibacterial soap on the side. I glanced at the collection of diplomas and the tiny chair meant for me. My disbelief withered. My insecurity grew. And tears started to form.

The nurse might have been thirty years old, maybe younger. By the time she had the blood-pressure cuff up my arm, tears were weighing heavily on my lower eyelids. One at a time at first, they rolled down my cheek. Soon, several at a time were rolling, and finally, whole collections fell in clumps onto the book in my lap.

And with the tears came a torrent of words. I told the nurse that I'd had only a little tingling in my hands, that it wasn't painful and couldn't be permanent. That it couldn't be multiple sclerosis. I told her that Dr. Silver thought it was multiple sclerosis but that it had to be something else.

"Tingling is annoying, isn't it?" she said, and told me that her boyfriend had to add padding to the seat of her Harley because her feet fell asleep. Bewildered, I kept crying. She got the numbers she needed off my arm, wrote them down, and rolled the cuff up and put it away.

She had me step on the scale. Even with my shoes on, I weighed only 115. I'm five foot six and had weighed 120 since college. "What?" I said. "I can't be one fifteen. Do you think that's the steroids?"

"Probably," she said. "How long you been on them?"

"Five days."

"You're lucky. Most people gain weight on them. One woman put on thirty pounds in a week."

"Good God, she must have been able to watch herself expanding."

The nurse put down the folder she was holding and reached for the door. She looked at me and saw that I was still crying. "At least you're not in Oncology," she said. "The doctor will be with you in a minute."

*At least I'm not in Oncology? Really?*

By the time Silver came in, my tears were dry and I had gone back to the book. I said hello and pulled out my legal pad. He took a seat on the stool near the examining table and opened a folder the nurse left behind.

"How are you feeling?" he asked. "I'm glad you decided not to go to India."

"Look, I've got a lot of questions," I said, launching in. I asked if any of the chemicals recently added to my system—the vaccines, the antibiotics, the steroids or some combination of those—could have anything to do with the tingling.

Silver ignored the question and, like the nurse, tried to explain how much worse life could be.

"It's like a bell curve," he said. "Two percent of the population that has MS never has any symptoms worse than what you have now."

"Hmm" was all I managed to say. I had asked about drugs I'd taken, and he ignored my question so completely that I felt like I hadn't said anything at all. I didn't know how to say, "Wait, you didn't answer my question." I had said some variation of that hundreds of times professionally, but personally, in this scary sterile room, I was at a loss.

Perhaps the steroids were wreaking havoc with my concentration *and* my determination. Or maybe the disconnect between my questions and his answer, my assumption of kindness and his absolute lack of it, were too big to reconcile in the moment. Same for the gap between how I was feeling and the severity of the diagnosis.

That was what seemed strangest—the gap between what my body was telling me and what Silver was saying. I was sitting in a neurologist's office, on the ninth floor of some building where people go to get growths removed, organs replaced and cancer radiated, and I felt good. My body felt better than good. My mind, on the other hand, was beyond bonkers—doing doughnuts like a Corvette on ice—but my physical strength and stamina were the same as always. I could have darted out the door, down the hall, down the stairs and out the front doors toward City Park. I could have run a 10K if I had to, not with blinding speed but at a respectable one-hour interval. Nothing hurt, all my body parts moved as directed and my mind was sharp as always—or would have been without the panic and Prednisone. The tingling was still in my fingertips and now a bit in my toes, but it seemed relatively minor, like a secret I should have kept and allowed to quietly slink away.

And I wished I had looked for answers myself instead of calling people on my insurance company's roster and expecting them to fix me. I wish I had Googled "tingling" or called a series of experts to see what it might mean, told them I was a reporter on a story. I wish I had dosed myself with vitamin B to see what that did, or had tried anything at all to have avoided this meeting with Silver and the one before it.

And yet, despite all my wishes, despite all the woulda-shoulda-couldas I knew were irrelevant, here I was, sitting in a teeny exam room with a professorial-looking man in a white lab coat. He tilted his head to the side, and his blue eyes looked weary, as if I were a nagging problem to be solved.

I shook it off and moved to my next question. What about vitamin D? Should we check my levels on that? I'd read it was related to both nerve health and the immune system. And how about vitamin

B12? The Mayo Clinic says a deficiency leads to tingling and, if left untreated, other neurological problems.

I had questions about the probiotics I had started taking to ready my digestive system for whatever I encountered in India.

Silver agreed to order a vitamin D test and said the probiotics probably wouldn't hurt. No word on the B12.

I wanted an answer and yet didn't push for one. As frustrated as I was, I stayed polite because I thought I needed this guy. I thought he was on my side. I was afraid if I asked the wrong question, he might refuse to answer, or worse, he might answer with something I didn't want to know. He might dig deeper and find something even worse than MS. I held back on the follow-up questions. He moved to the edge of his chair like he was ready to go, like his time was limited and more valuable than mine. Like his answers were final.

But I wasn't done. Even though I was on the verge of tears again, I finally, *finally* tapped into a bit of muscle memory from my reporting days. I had a lot to ask and a lot to say. I shifted forward in my seat, willing him to sit back in his.

"Steroids," I said. "Everything flies faster on them."

I told Silver how they busted up my meditation practice, how I couldn't quiet my monkey mind no matter what. I told him how the night before I'd had a craving for a spinach salad, only more serious than usual.

"I told the waitress, 'I need a spinach salad without bacon and I need it now or someone's going to get hurt.'"

For the first time, Silver's expression changed. He smiled and said that, yes, that happens.

I asked about the weight loss. I'd lost five pounds in five days. This was not a promising development.

"Yes," Silver said, "this happens sometimes."

"I don't understand how this could be MS. If the tingling's caused by a permanent problem in my brain, why would it come and go so easily? I feel better after getting a massage or practicing yoga."

He shook his head. "Yes, of course. Doesn't matter."

*Really? Something that makes me feel better doesn't matter? It matters to me.* And yet again, I didn't pursue it. He had said what he said, with authority, as if that solved that. I pressed on.

The tingling had grown since I started taking the Prednisone. More intense in my hands, and it also landed in my toes. It seemed like this could be a good sign—the treatment for MS wasn't working so I probably didn't have MS. Or jacked up as I was on panic, Prednisone and faith in experts, it seemed equally likely that this was a terrible sign. Could it be that my condition was deteriorating so rapidly that even the drugs weren't stopping my slide? Remembering Joan's story, I held my breath. *Shit,* I thought. *I could be blind any moment and I drove here. How will I get home?*

My mind raced through all these questions and concerns in a nanosecond, and yet when I opened my mouth, I asked only why I felt worse on the Prednisone.

"It could take a while for the drug to work through your system," Silver said. "It may take a while to get going and it continues in your system for a while, weeks, maybe a month, after you stop taking it. Prednisone behaves differently in different bodies."

*Why, then, hand it out like candy?* I thought. And more important, why did I down those little pills like they were just sugary tablets from a Pez dispenser? And why continue to take them? I took the first handful because I figured Silver prescribed a specific dose for a reason and knew what he was doing. Then, on the info sheet the pharmacist gave me, buried in the small print, I read that failing to take the entire prescription could lead to suicidal tendencies. Having limited experience with doctors and less with drugs, I gave the pharmacist similar respect. I didn't think she would hand out papers that were meant to be ignored.

*Great, these things are making me lose weight, chew out well-intending waitresses and second-guess every waking thought. What could be worse? If I stop taking them, and contemplate suicide, that would be worse, of course.*

Finally, I asked Silver the biggest question: "Doesn't the *M* stand for multiple, in that there have to be multiple episodes over time and space?"

The doctor shook his head. "Well," he said, as if sticking to the definition like that was for amateurs. "The tingling has been going on for so long and there are enough lesions on your spinal cord that we can assume they were sequential, one after another, causing the continuous symptom."

He said it as he had said everything else: kindly, authoritatively and leaving little room for debate.

He made another move like he was getting up to go, and I looked back at the pad of paper in my lap. "And don't we have to rule out everything else?" I asked before he could stand.

"The blood tests did that," he said and moved on to talking about medication.

Silver sailed from "MS is the most likely explanation" to "You have MS—start medication" so swiftly and smoothly that I nearly went with him. He gave me four info sheets on each of the different drug protocols and suggested I read them. "I've been doing this for thirty years," he said. "So I have an opinion, but why don't you take a look and we'll discuss the different treatment options."

I asked again if he was sure about the diagnosis, and he said he was. "I've been doing this for thirty years," he repeated. "It's the most common diagnosis I give to women like you."

I must have had a question on my face, because he said, "Young and athletic."

*Haven't we gone through this already?* "I'm not that young."

"You're young enough," he said once more. "You can get a second opinion if you want. If you go to another doctor within the HMO, we'll pay for it. If you go outside the network, you're out of pocket."

When he used *we*, he didn't include me. *We* meant his team: the insurance company, his colleagues and him. I was the odd one out. They were "we" and I was diseased.

"I know I'm overwhelmed right now and I'm going to have many more questions," I said. "Who do I call?"

"You call me," Silver said.

I thought I misunderstood. He seemed so busy and unable to engage in conversation even when I was sitting in front of him. "Isn't there a nurse or someone who answers calls and questions?"

"No," he said. "You call me."

I don't have much of a poker face. And I was surprised.

Silver caught it. "I'm busy," he said, "and I don't answer my phone. If you leave a message, I'll call you back within twenty-four hours. I don't like to have conversations by email, but if you send me a note saying you want to talk to me, that you have a question, I'll call you back within twenty-four hours."

He said this emphatically. I believed him.

## CHAPTER 5

# SNAKES AND LADDERS

Day six on the Prednisone and I couldn't sit still. I couldn't get warm and couldn't stop my mind from racing through the scariest scenarios. Most involved wheelchairs. Some included full-blown, four-limbed paralysis. And while my body stayed stationery in these scenes, my mind sprinted around itself and around the room and around the world as if it knew that someday it would be the only part of me that could run. After a lifetime of globe-trotting and marathon-running, my body wouldn't be able to.

I inhaled to prevent a big cry, then gave in and cried away. I sat on the floor and sobbed. I rolled over and lay face down on the hardwood and sobbed some more.

Eventually, I was cried out. Truly, I had no more tears. I got off the floor and went into the kitchen.

I had the four one-pagers that Silver gave me on each of the drug protocols, and even though the sight of them fortified the fear and sadness that seemed to be all around me, I made a pot of peppermint tea and forced my mind to focus and my eyes to read.

The options included different brands of interferon drugs, the same drugs Joan had told me about. I sat on the oversized couch and started with the first section on the first page: "How the Drug Works." On each page, the header was followed by the same sentence: "The way Rebif works on MS is not clear."

Thinking I must be missing something—no self-respecting communications pro would headline a section "How the Drug Works" only to follow it with the equivalent of "we have no idea"—I flipped through the pages a few times to be sure that's what they were saying. And they were. As if the drafters of these documents figured no one would read these things or that anyone who did would be too afraid to question their logic, they wrote: "The way Copaxone works on MS is not clear," "The way Betaseron works on MS is not clear," and "The way Avonex works on MS is not clear."

I was scared but not scared enough to tinker with my brain chemistry without knowing why. I kept reading and kept seeing more inconsistencies and coming up with more questions.

Three of the four pages said the drugs "work against viruses and stimulate the immune system." My confidence sank further. Silver said that MS was an autoimmune condition, and that my immune system was on overdrive, attacking my nervous system. If that were the case, why stimulate it and push it to work even harder? It sounded like a recipe for disaster.

The next section referred to different types of the disease—relapsing-remitting and secondary-progressive. Silver never told me which kind he thought I had or how anyone could tell the difference. He just said I had MS and should take drugs.

I forced myself to read the section titled "Studies." Each pharmaceutical company studied its drug with sample sizes of 251 people, 301 people, 372 people and 560 people, respectively.

*That's all you've got? I've got more Facebook friends than any of these studies. And who* are *these people?* The info sheets didn't say if they were men or women, young or old, how many lesions they had, or their range of symptoms. Were they in wheelchairs, or did they have slight tingling sensations in their fingertips? Were they like me? Would anyone with a slight tingling sign up for a drug trial when the company couldn't explain how the drug worked?

And for the fourth time in as many minutes, I wished I'd never told anyone about the tingling. The pins and needles were never painful, just annoying, and until I took the Prednisone, the tingling was limited to very small body parts, just fingertips. And in comparison, this experience—reading these pages—was excruciating. Still, I continued.

All four drug companies used the same language on results. Each said that patients on the drug, whichever drug it was, "had about one-third fewer flares than patients with no medication."

Four drug tests presumably done in four separate locations for four separate drug companies all landed in the exact same spot, or "about" the same spot, on the one-third mark.

"This is bullshit," I said out loud. A coincidence like this—four studies landing on the exact same depressing dime?—it's impossible. And ridiculous. I knew a bit about cherry-picking data. Over and over, I'd seen political consultants pick apart and manipulate polling data so they could say a majority of the population approved of whatever candidate or cause they were selling. And pharmaceutical companies—a $700 billion industry—had much more to gain or lose than any political spin doctor.

I had no doubt the drug companies presented only the best data they had and "about one-third" was it. That just wasn't going to cut it for me.

"How do they get away with this?" I asked no one in particular.

I flipped to the back side of each page to read the potential side effects. These included injection-site reaction (inflammation, pain or rash in as many as 85 percent of patients), menstrual disorders, heart palpitations, chest pain, shortness of breath, flu-like symptoms (in as many as 75 percent of patients), depression or suicidal thoughts, a decrease in the number of white blood cells, and changes in liver enzymes. For the flu, depression and liver damage, the info sheets conveniently suggested ibuprofen, acetaminophen, antidepressants and lab tests every three months to check complete blood count and liver function. "Be sure to keep appointments," it read.

"Fuck all!" I yelled and grabbed my phone.

"Bruce," I cried as soon as he answered. "Silver gave me four pages on the four drugs and none of them work. They did studies on, like, two hundred and fifty-one people—why two fifty-one? Why not two fifty or three hundred or three thousand or some big number, or at least some even number? Do you think the extra forty-nine people died? Or something worse?"

Bruce almost snorted a small, uncomfortable laugh.

"And even with two hundred and fifty-one people, they proved nothing," I continued. "Patients on the drug had one-third fewer episodes than people without. That doesn't feel like enough to outweigh the risks. These things cause heart palpations, liver failure and suicidal tendencies. In most people. Eighty-five percent get the nasty impacts and only 'about one-third' see any benefit. So which is the side effect and which is the main effect?"

Worn out from my rant, I started sobbing. Again.

"Slow it down, Jody," Bruce said. "Wait a second, hang on."

I heard him moving to a quieter place. Poor guy, he was probably sitting in some bar on the beach in Cabo when I dialed.

"This doesn't sound right," he said. "You're not going to take those. This doesn't make sense. Why don't you give Christopher a call?"

A friend of Bruce's in Vancouver, Christopher had cured himself of Lyme disease, which was thought at the time to be permanent and incurable and is still considered difficult to treat if not caught right away. He spent years using diet and exercise to reverse the effects of Lyme on his own body, and he now served as a consultant for folks who didn't like a diagnosis or prognosis and wanted options. He helped people with any kind of condition sort out their diets and served as a conduit to other healing professionals—some alternative, some more mainstream.

As I listened to Bruce's voice, solid and sure, I started to relax. We talked a while longer, and slowly I started to feel more whole. And less alone.

When I felt calm enough to say good-bye, we hung up and I called Christopher. I introduced myself and told him the story up to that point, including the four drug protocols. He asked where I grew up and how industrial my home town was.

"I grew up in Detroit," I said.

"Oh," he said, and exhaled audibly. "And where do you live now?"

"Denver."

"Yeah," Christopher said. "There's a high occurrence of MS there."

He asked more questions, ones Silver had never asked. Christopher interviewed me the way I hope I interview people. His questions were open-ended and intended to learn about me as an individual. He avoided yes or no questions designed to slot someone quickly into a box or category like "young, athletic and female."

Christopher and I stayed on the phone for an hour or more. He seemed interested in helping, suggesting I come to Vancouver to meet with him and doctors he knew who could potentially help me decide how to proceed. Since I was still on stolen India time, I said I would for a couple of weeks. We settled on dates, and he asked me to fax or email all my test results to him.

"No problem," I said and hung up, thinking that just getting out of town and into new scenery would be helpful. And I loved the idea of having someone to help me navigate. I knew I needed support more than ever before.

Next up, I called Sanoviv, the holistic hospital in Mexico that Jonathan's friend Joan suggested. I spoke to a doctor named Harmony, who told me about herself (she studied functional medicine in Mexico, had two kids, was thirty-four) and about their program of integrated medical care. Sanoviv patients see a kinesiologist to test muscle strength, nutritionists to evaluate diet, a psychologist to explore emotional components of an illness, and a physician to oversee and coordinate the entire program. Individually, each member of the team evaluates the patient, and the team as a whole meets to plot the treatment phase, which in my case Harmony said would most likely involve the neuro-repair program of a high dosage of vitamin C, time in a hyperbaric chamber, and massage and detoxifying body wraps. Each day would include treatments, meditation sessions, delicious, healthy meals and an ocean view. Twenty-one days for $22,000.

I kept looking.

The next day, and every day after that, I forced myself into a routine. I'd wake up, brush my teeth, light a candle and sit on a cushion on the floor in the middle of the room to meditate. This too was a gift from Bruce.

Early on, when I was visiting him on Pender Island, in British Columbia, for the first time, he had patted me high on the chest one day and said, "Babe, you breathe way up here. Can you relax?"

When I looked at him with confusion—I didn't know there was any other way to breathe—he took my hand, stood up off the couch and guided me to a seat on the floor in front of a statue of the Buddha. The statue sat before an enormous picture window that faced south, looking out over the water and far into the background, to Mount Rainier.

Bruce lit a stick of incense and said, "Sweetie, you have to learn to breathe. Meditation will help you. It helped me. Just slow it down, focus on your breathing, breathe with me."

And then we did. For a while. Long slow inhales and longer, slower exhales. We sat breathing together, inhaling as one and filling up on each other's energy until we couldn't not touch each other anymore. Then we made love right there on the floor and eventually moved to the couch. Maybe it was the big orgasms that followed my first meditation session that glued me to the practice. Or maybe not. Either way, I'd been practicing daily since then.

Most days I found the practice calming. Now, though, when I sat, I found it hard to stop the lousy cycle of scary questions about my health. At forty-three years old, I was scared and wanted mothering. But I didn't feel like there was anyone I could ask for that, definitely not my mom. Through most of my adult life (and probably back into childhood too) when I faced difficult situations or stressful choices, including my mother in them only increased the level of difficulty.

College graduation, for example, was stressful. I had no career plan and a mountain of debt. My father came to the graduation ceremonies, and my mother was furious that he was there. (My parents had divorced when I was twenty.) She was equally livid when I got married. Not that she didn't like my husband; she did. She loved him and was angry with me anyway for reasons she couldn't articulate and I never understood. Then, when my husband and I threw a dinner party to celebrate our relationship, my mom was outraged. Our friends brought gifts and stood to toast our happiness. My mom sat quietly throughout and called a few days later to tell me she was disappointed. "It just wasn't enough," she said.

And finally, and maybe hilariously if you're anyone other than me, my mother wound herself up to another stratospheric level of rage when I decided to get divorced. "You're jumping off a cliff. I won't stand for it," she thundered into my voice mail. We didn't talk for months.

Needless to say, my mom wasn't someone I turned to in a crisis. Whatever was going on in my body, I wasn't going to tell her. The diagnosis was difficult enough. And at this point, she thought I was in India and I had no need to tell her otherwise. Same with my sister.

My father, however, was another story. While my mom remarried straight away, my father never did, and over the years, we developed a loving father-daughter relationship.

In his sixties, my dad was diagnosed with diabetes. I was living in New York at the time, and once he was diagnosed, he waited until his next visit to tell me about it. We went to Katz's, an old-school deli that opened its doors in 1888. The place still had signs on the wall from World War II—"Send a Salami to your boy in the Army"—and waiters who probably started working around the same time.

My dad tested the remains of his Yiddish with the waiter and ordered a Dr. Brown's Cel-Ray soda and a pastrami sandwich for lunch. I ordered eggs. We talked about the Yankees, President Clinton, and whether George Pataki could get reelected as governor. When the plates were cleared, my dad told me he'd seen a doctor. First, he said, he'd lost a lot of weight then had to urinate all the time. The doctor ran blood tests and declared it diabetes.

He finished the story and ordered pie for dessert.

On a night in early January, years past his diabetes diagnosis and days past Silver's diagnosis of me, I called my dad. He was surprised to hear from me. I told him I canceled my trip and the reason. He stayed quiet and listened. I told him that I didn't believe the diagnosis and that I was going to go to Vancouver to seek other opinions.

"Do you want me to come?" he asked.

In his seventies then, my father still practiced law. He was prepared to clear his calendar for two weeks to spend time with me in Vancouver. I was touched. And surprised. That might be what normal families do for each other—or it may be my fantasy of normal—yet I didn't expect it.

"No, no," I said. "That's OK. I'll be there for two weeks. If I get there and I want you to come, I'll call and let you know."

"Are you going to be in a hospital?"

"No, I'm staying at a friend's place, and I'm seeing a number of specialists."

We talked a while longer and I told him I'd call from Vancouver. I went to sleep happy that I had talked to my dad and glad to know that he was there and that he understood.

In the morning, I considered who else I would tell. Friends were tricky. I still didn't feel like I knew the story, how anyone would react or what questions they would ask. Lauren's comment still stung: "He's fine. He gets around OK. He has a guy who lifts him out of bed in the morning."

JD was an unknown. A friend of a friend whom I'd met a few years earlier, JD and I liked each other and weren't particularly close. Not knowing I was supposed to be in India or about to go to Vancouver, he emailed me in early January and we made a date for lunch.

By the day we met, I had finished taking the steroids. I was feeling more optimistic about the whole prognosis and was taking ownership of my health—looking at other resources and reviewing my options. And physically, the morning we were to meet, I felt great. The tingling was down to a minimum, back to where it was pre-steroids, and the sun was shining and my energy surging. I wasn't sure how much I was going to tell JD, if anything. I figured I'd know when I saw him.

A little before one o'clock, I walked around the block to the restaurant. When I was within twenty yards of JD, the tingling kicked up, creeping up my arms from my hands and making itself known in my feet.

*Interesting*, I thought. I wondered what caused it. We hugged and I felt awkward.

The restaurant was closed, so we walked a couple blocks to another. We got to the second restaurant and sat down on the clunky wooden chairs, and I felt a new sensation, a tingling centered on a spot in my low back and firing down both legs, not unbearable but definitely distracting.

I took note of it and wondered whether this was temporary or if this was the start of something permanent. I pictured Joan going blind and heard Silver saying he didn't know how the disease would progress. Anything could be a symptom, and any feeling could be a warning sign of something awful and sudden.

As I wondered about this, I tried to shake off my fear of the future and stay in the present. *Stay right here, right now, right here, right now*, I told myself. I tried to note without judgment what I was feeling and to focus on my friend and our conversation.

The conversation, however, was dark. JD had left his most recent girlfriend and although he talked about saying good-bye as if she were someone he knew from the office—"There was nothing wrong, we just couldn't work out the logistics"—he seemed pretty down about it.

At the moment, I was concerned for him and worried about me. The more we talked, the more the gently distracting pins-and-needles feeling morphed into a high-volume prickly sensation that started in my lower back and demanded attention. I considered panicking. I took a breath and noted what was happening.

Eventually, we paid our bill and stepped outside into a gorgeous Colorado day. The sunlight clashed with our gloomy lunch. We hugged and JD jumped on his bike and pedaled north.

I started walking the two blocks south to my house. As I crossed the street, I noticed that everything was calming down. A half block later, the tingling retreated all the way back into my extremities, just fingers and a touch in my toes. When I stepped inside my house and sat down on the couch, everything was as it had been before I went out. Relieved to feel closer to normal again, I was also strangely fascinated that the physical sensations could come and go so quickly, seemingly dependent on emotions that were neither mine nor spoken out loud.

I emailed Joan right away and told her the story. "Do you think lesions on the spinal cord create a kind of superpower?"

"Yes," she wrote back. "We have a lot in common."

She and I didn't get to talk about it so I don't know what she meant or if she could explain how it worked. My friend Joe, however, came through when I told him about it. "Wow, forget MS," he said. "You're like a human mood ring."

✚ ✚ ✚

That night, I dreamt of a snake. He was a pale, earthy tone from tip to tail, and I was not afraid. He sat coiled and quiet right at my feet and seemed to belong right where he was. He held my gaze with his and never wavered as he slowly started growing taller, rocking slowly, methodically, almost imperceptibly, right and left, right and left. When his head reached the height of my belly button, he silently and smoothly veered left and wound his way over my hip and around to my back.

In the dream, I was translucent. I could see through my skin to watch as he started at the base of my spine and began winding his way up, the way a snake slowly, luxuriously, winds its way around something straight and true. When he had wrapped all the way up my spine and his head was circling my neck, he continued out in front of me and turned back to face me.

We were face-to-face, nearly nose-to-nose, and I was still unafraid. I don't think he spoke. He may have. Or he may have let me know wordlessly. Either way, when I was looking into his eyes, I understood: we are in this together.

We held each other's gaze a while longer, and the snake made sure I understood: we are in this together.

I woke the next morning knowing I was going to find the answer. Whatever was going on in my body, I was going to be OK and the answer would be found inside me. Different parts of me needed to weave their way back together perhaps, but there was nothing in me that did not belong and nothing I needed that I didn't already have.

In other words, there was nothing to add and nothing to remove.

I decided I could become calm and leave all the chaos on the outside. I could distance myself from the noise coming from Silver and Joan, the med tech in the MRI room, the nurse in Silver's office, and anyone else who was telling me about *me*, insisting that I was damaged and had to follow directions to stay still.

Inside, I was whole and complete and perfectly healthy, if only a little disconnected.

*We are in this together.* The snake in my dream was me, or a subconscious part of me talking to me, saying, "We are in this together. Trust me."

And, as if to make sure I trusted him (or perhaps trusted myself), the snake made sure I saw him again and again. After my morning meditation, I made some tea, ate breakfast and went to my office to continue researching drug treatments. As I clicked on the American Medical Association's home page, I saw a snake wrapped around a spine. It's the rod of Asclepius, the Greek god of healing, the website explained, and it evokes the serpent-entwined staff that Moses lifted in the book of Exodus: everyone who looked upon it was healed.

*Everyone who looked upon it was healed.*

Holy shit.

In the afternoon, I went to a yoga studio to stretch with other people. The instructor, a beautiful woman with dirty blond hair, started talking about *Kundalini*—a Sanskrit word that means "coiled," like a snake. "*Kundalini* energy," she said, "sits dormant, coiled at the base of your spine. And when you are ready to awaken, she rises and travels up and around your spine, lighting up each chakra."

I walked home feeling the usual post-yoga calm and something more than that. I felt quietly energized, ready to climb, one rung at a time if I had to, back to better health. I was almost eager to see what I was made of, to understand the inner workings of me.

CHAPTER 6

# OH SO RADICAL

As the plane made its final descent, Vancouver sparkled just out the window, just off the wing, as it always does. A gorgeous city, surrounded by water and sky, it looked, smelled and felt like love to me. I'd never been before I met Bruce, and since then, I'd gone every couple of months to see him. As undefined as our relationship was, he and his city were irresistible to me.

I walked off the plane and through the familiar airport, smiling past the indigenous waterfowl display and listening to the recorded whistling and cooing. I always found those staccato chirps both silly and soothing, like I was entering an exotic new world, a playful place just waiting to be explored. And on this trip, more than most, I was exploring.

Back in Denver, before takeoff, and before the snake dream, I was a small, trembling girl terrified that the feeling in my fingertips was a sure sign, as Silver said, of horrible things to come. Hopped up on steroids, I curled in on myself to shield myself against an awful future. A few hours at altitude always delivered a complete change of attitude, however. I was a whole new me: optimistic, confident and marching into adventure; looking for information in a sunny, sparkling, cosmopolitan piece of Canada. The tingling feeling was still there, but its significance seemed less certain.

In my reporting days, every flight led to a new collection of characters, a new story line and a brand-new chance to get it right. If the last story wasn't good, or even if it was an outright disaster, catching a flight meant leaving it behind and getting ready to tackle another. I felt the same way now, although I was on my own assignment, searching for clues to gain a better understanding of my health so I could write a happier ending.

The birds chirped and people flowed onto the moving sidewalk. I breezed by the whole scene and strode the length of the airport, past dozens of gates and sleepy crowds waiting to leave. Along the way, smiling volunteers in Vancouver 2010 golf shirts said hello and asked, "Can I direct you toward the credentialing tables?" No, not this time. I didn't need credentials. The Vancouver Olympics were only weeks away, and journalists were starting to arrive. I wasn't one of them. I didn't need to sign in or find a bus to the press center.

I needed information, that's all. And not just a little bit—I had that. I wanted a wealth of information, a diversity of opinions and ideas.

I walked the switchback lines to the customs agent, had the usual chat—"vacation," "staying with a friend," "thank you, sir"—and grabbed my bag off the carousel. I found Terry waiting among the limo drivers holding name cards just beyond the glass doors.

A tall, gentle guy in his early thirties, Terry was a friend of Bruce's sons. He became part of the family and had ultimately started working for Bruce. As far as I could tell, his job was doing whatever Bruce needed, asked or suggested. In the time I'd known them, Terry picked me up at the airport a handful of times, worked on Bruce's house on Pender Island, and spent six months in India when Bruce suggested he learn to meditate. This time he was there because Bruce was still away on business. He'd be joining me later—and I couldn't wait to see him.

Six feet tall with an easy smile, Terry is friendly and sweet in a such a pure way that it's hard to imagine that he spent years living a more dangerous and mistrustful life. Tattoos over his arms and back are souvenirs from that era. "You look great," he said, giving me a speedy hug. "You look like you've lost weight."

"Yeah, I've been sick," I said.

I can be a real downer at times.

Terry took my luggage to the black Range Rover (Bruce's, of course) and opened the door for me. As we left the airport, I told him about the diagnosis. He knew someone with MS and said she seemed to be doing OK. I told him about the steroids and how they made me crazy, that they made me lose weight. "That's weird," he said. "Guys at the gym take 'em to put on pounds."

Terry drove me to Bruce's apartment, a beautiful three-bedroom place with floor-to-ceiling windows in the living room and kitchen. I could sit at the counter, enjoy a cup of tea, and watch sailboats bobbing in the harbor and runners jogging to Stanley Park.

The master bedroom, at the end of the long hall, was warm and cozy. On top of a tall, dark wooden bureau, there was a large glass plate on a stand. Two and a half feet across, the blown glass had hundreds of soft brown Buddhas sitting in concentric circles. When I lit the candles behind it, Buddhas danced around the room.

The bed was luxury-resort comfy, and when I pulled the drapes, the room was dark as a deep cave—perfect for a solid sleep. Just looking around, I knew I was going to have one of those nights in which I'd nod out as soon as the covers landed on my chest. I'd wake in the exact same position, fully rested, ten or eleven hours later—something my mixed-up body desperately needed.

In the bathroom, there was a wonderfully deep tub with an assortment of candles and a separate glass-walled shower. Given that I hadn't gone to the Quiet Healing Center in India because of this mysterious illness, and given all that had transpired since I canceled that trip, this place felt like a lovely second choice. It felt safe. I felt like I could breathe here.

My optimism was so sweet and strong that all of Vancouver seemed to be on my side. When Terry left, I walked outside and for the first time in what felt like months, the fog lifted from my brain and I saw the world in clear detail again. I saw people smiling and laughing. There were Japanese noodle shops and warm Italian restaurants, a store with high-end bikes and others with trendy shoes and cashmere sweaters. There were people everywhere, and all of us were an easy walk from the water, where the boats were bobbing in their slips.

I walked into the grocery store, and a woman handed me something warm and yummy to taste. Another woman, when I realized I had only American dollars, said, "No problem, I can convert it for ya. Do you want change in Canadian or U.S.? Should probably have some Canadian, right?"

As I walked back toward the apartment, I was grateful for this temporary sanctuary in the West End of Vancouver. And I was grateful that my nervous system was calming down. I felt like I'd been on speed since the MRI, and now, finally—*finally*—I could take a moment, take a breath and figure out what was happening. I was ready to learn about my health and work to regain it, with someone who had a different perspective.

And Christopher certainly had a different perspective from Dr. Silver in Denver. And a different, more animated demeanor.

A tall, skinny guy with dark hair, Christopher looked like he could spring forward at any moment, like a runner off the blocks. "MS is generally a bullshit diagnosis," he said immediately upon meeting me. "It's a catchall that doctors say when they don't know what else is going on. What did the neurologist tell you about it?"

I told him that Silver didn't say much definitively: he didn't know the cause, although he thought it had something to do with chicken pox; he didn't know how it would affect my body or how the drugs he suggested might work.

"Right," Christopher said. "The only thing they know for certain is that it's forever. If they diagnose MS and it goes away, then it must have been a misdiagnosis, which means they'd have made a mistake. It's bullshit."

"Wait," I said. "You mean they know so little about it that one set of symptoms can 'definitely' be MS until the symptoms go away and then they 'definitely weren't' MS?"

"Yeah, right. It's a moving target and let's not worry about the label anyway," he said. "I'm not a doctor, I'm not a naturopath and I'm not a licensed practitioner in health. I'm an educator in the field of holistic health and I'll share information that changed my life. I'll give you information so you can act on it if it feels right to you. And it is up to you," he said. "Most people don't know what feels right to them. They just do as they're told."

*Do as they're told?* I wondered. That's not exactly my strong suit. In college when everyone encouraged me to do internships and prepare for a career, I studied philosophy, worked in kitchens and taught canoeing in the summers. After school, conventional wisdom said I should start working at small newspapers and work my way up to bigger and bigger publications. I took jobs at the racetrack and applied to *Sports Illustrated* instead.

Christopher and I were still standing near the door, so I invited him in. We took seats at the table near the windows overlooking the water. He was ready to share his wisdom, and as a recovering reporter, I was ready to take it all down. For the first time in a while, with a notebook on the table and a pen in my hand, I felt back in my element, ready to do what I'd always done to make sense of the world and to feel safe. I'd ask questions, lots of questions, and relentlessly gather information without judging any of it. Somewhere deep inside, I knew the world was beautifully complex, that at any given moment there were a number of right answers to the same question, several solutions to a single problem. Looking back, this was one reason I became a journalist in the first place. I collected information and reported every story from endless angles just to make sure the world outside matched the truth I believed on the inside.

And in this case, I needed to report out the story so there could be more answers and so I could make sure I found the right one, regardless of what that was. I didn't want Silver's diagnosis to stand all alone, with nothing to compare it to, no data before or after that point in time, no idea how it fit into any pattern. I needed to ask dozens of questions to put the tingling sensation and Silver's take on it into context, so I could see options and possibilities that I hadn't seen before. So I launched into full-on reporter mode.

Subconsciously, I knew that as long as I was in reporter mode, I couldn't be in sick-person mode. In other words, I couldn't let myself be a sick person.

I asked Christopher how he got started in the healing educator business. He started the tale in 1986, when he had a successful photography business in Vancouver. All was going well, so well that he decided to put work on hold and tour Australia for six months. When he returned to Canada, he was exhausted and had a fever. It lasted a while, so he saw a doctor, who told him, "It's mono. Get some rest."

A few months later, feeling worse, Christopher went to another doctor who said it was Epstein-Barr virus. This time the prescription was, "Eat well. Get some rest." For the next four years, he ate well, rested, and felt worse and worse.

"There was no diagnosis that led to a practical treatment," he said. "I had all the symptoms of MS—arthritis, palsy and heart problems, but no lesions. I saw several doctors who said nothing was wrong, take antidepressants."

At first this confused me further. Christopher had had horrible MS-like symptoms—but he had no lesions, and so somehow he received no diagnosis. I, on the other hand, had lesions and comparatively minor symptoms. But it was the lesions the neurologist latched onto, and it was his interpretation of them that had sent me spiraling downward in fear.

Christopher made a pot of peppermint tea and told me that, eventually, a friend of his who had similar symptoms was diagnosed with Lyme disease. Christopher went back to his doctor and suggested they look for Lyme. When the test came back positive, he received intravenous antibiotics.

Still, the symptoms persisted. "There were four years of relapses and remissions because the antibiotics never cured the cause," Christopher said. "The antibiotics killed it in my blood but not in my central nervous system because they don't cross the blood-brain barrier."

Finally, he suffered the rock-bottom relapse. The pain was so great and the fear so intense that he thought to himself, "I cannot live like this."

He contemplated going back for another round of intravenous antibiotics and stopped himself. "Isn't doing the same thing and expecting different results the definition of insanity?" he wondered.

(Good point.) And then he remembered something he'd learned in a Tony Robbins seminar. The international self-help star was speaking about success in business, and the sentiment worked here too: don't go to a teacher; find someone who's successfully doing what you want to do and copy them.

Instead of seeking yet another physician who could talk about symptoms from a safe distance, Christopher started to hunt for folks who had experienced his same symptoms—people who had been submerged in them, felt like they were drowning in them—and then had managed to successfully swim away. In other words, he looked for people who left degenerative diseases behind by taking control of their own health. He found many of these people in health-food stores.

Suddenly, I realized that I felt the best I had felt in months. Somewhere between Denver and this moment, the tingling had left my hands and settled uncomfortably into a spot between my toes, like I was wearing flip-flops (except I wasn't). But to me, it wasn't the physical sensation, the tingling, that was a big deal. It was what Silver said the sensation implied: that I had a degenerative neurological disease. Christopher quickly dismissed the whole doomsday outlook. (Maybe it was his hopeful demeanor that caused the tingling to recede—since I had become a human mood ring and all.)

At that moment, talking intensely with a near stranger in this stunning apartment, I also realized I wanted to follow his path. I wanted to know people who didn't take on a strange diagnosis as a life sentence. If my MRI had shown lesions, I wanted to know that that didn't mean disaster was necessarily looming, and I wanted to know how I could take control of it instead of letting it sink me. I needed a role model, and this friend of Bruce's, this tall, skinny guy, he was it.

"They were talking about the weird world of natural healings, and it was very confusing to me," Christopher said of the folks he met early in his journey. "This one said buffered vitamin C and that one said natural vitamin C. This one said reverse osmosis and another said filtered water. It all seemed contradictory."

Pain can be a powerful motivator, and Christopher was sick and tired of being, well, sick and tired. Despite the contradictions, he searched for commonalities. Themes emerged. He kept studying, and over time, he put together an eight-piece plan for optimal health: breathe, hydrate, move, stop the poisons, take out the garbage, nourish, sleep and believe.

"These are the eight steps toward dynamic life and health," he said. "I say 'toward' because the potential is so huge."

Christopher explained how the eight ideas work together, serving as a platform for optimal health. I had questions about stopping the poisons and flushing them out of my system, and he was happy to answer. "It's important for the body to eliminate what it doesn't need," he said.

We talked about the effects of "new" toxins, like pesticides, herbicides, industrial fertilizers, fluoridated water and mercury fillings—new in the sense that until recently, people did not live with these things. As a species, we hadn't had time to adapt to and evolve around them. In labs, Christopher said, evolutionary biologists study fruit flies because the scientists can see the beginnings of the slightest hint of the idea of an adaptation after five hundred or six hundred generations. And fruit flies being busy, this all happens inside of a month.

Us humans, we go slow. We are only two or three generations away from the beginning of industrial agriculture, when scores of chemicals were introduced into our world and our food supply. The human body wasn't ready then, and we haven't adapted yet.

"The liver wasn't designed for the new chemicals we add to the environment," Christopher said. "So the body stores toxins in fat and connective tissue, waiting for the liver to catch up and deal with the toxins, but the liver is busy with food. So the toxins just stay there."

Fat cells serve as deep storage in a human body. When the body wants to tuck something out of the way, the way we might throw junk we don't want in the attic or a public storage space, the body dumps its junk in fat cells. With me, for whatever reason—good diet, good genes or just good luck—I've never carried a lot of fat on my body. The one place, however, that even the skinniest among us has fat cells is in our brains—fat cells comprise 60 percent of the brain—and the myelin sheath that coats the spinal cord. If my body was looking for a place to hide toxins, the central nervous system might have looked like a good place for the secret stash. Is that what the MRI showed? Mercury-made lesions?

Christopher had started reading the medical literature and studying how the body works nearly two decades earlier. And he was sharing his knowledge with me. I didn't ask him to cough up the citations or provide the original research any more than I asked Silver to show evidence that steroids stunt the immune system or that they were a good idea in my case.

We talked for hours until we were both exhausted. We walked around the corner to the Whole Foods store, each bought a juice and called it a day.

The next morning, after a deep, motionless sleep—not the anticipated eleven hours, but a solid nine—I stretched and sat down to meditate. I lit a candle before me on the floor and the one behind the glass plate. As I inhaled, I silently said, *So*, and on the exhales, *Hum. So hum, so hum.* It's so simple, and it means "I am that." I sat focusing on my breath, silently *so-humming* with the Buddhas dancing all around. After twenty minutes, I expressed gratitude, as I always did, for this life, this love, this mind, this body, this healing and all my teachers, in this and every present moment. *And, I'm grateful*, I added, *for this apartment. It's so sweet.*

An hour later, Christopher picked me up to go to a holistic healing center in the tony Yaletown neighborhood. There we met Daniel Smith, a health detective of sorts who studied nutrition, acupuncture and other therapies before opening the healing center. Tall and thin with gray hair, Daniel spoke gently and guided Christopher and I down the narrow hallway to his office—which was half the size of the office where Rebecca and I sat with Silver that awful day, yet so much more comfortable.

"Electroacupuncture according to Voll, or EAV," Daniel said, to introduce an odd machine that sat on his desk. It looked like the mini flight panel of an old airplane with its art-deco dials and needles and nobs.

"A German doctor named Voll created it in the 1950s," he said. "It measures the resistance of the skin at the acupuncture point. The optimum reading is fifty and there are six hundred points on the body that correspond to organs. It's a very simple, reliable test to determine your overall health by measuring energy levels at specific acupuncture points."

I didn't know much about acupuncture but was open to it since I'd once had a great experience back in New York to combat allergies. After trying all the over-the-counter allergy medicines that one sneezy spring, I was at the end of my rope and would have tried anything. A friend suggested acupuncture and gave me a name to call. I booked one session, sat with the needles in for half an hour and haven't suffered hay fever since. Even the acupuncturist was surprised.

Daniel handed me a small copper-colored rod to hold and took out a small penlike wand, both attached by wire to the EAV machine. I took off my shoes and socks, and he set about touching the wand to thirty-four points on my hands and another twenty on my feet. He watched the needle on the machine, and as he called out each number, Christopher wrote them down.

Most of the numbers were in the sweet spot around fifty—meaning that energy was flowing easily through the point. If a spot was too low or too high, it signaled an imbalance or obstruction. Three were mighty low: the right-eye lymphatic system was twenty, and the point that corresponds to hormonal activity was twenty-six. The pancreas was nineteen.

"Help me out here," I said. "My lymphatic system? My pancreas? I'm not sure I know what they do or what that means."

"Oh, right," Daniel said. "I can explain. The lymphatic system is the body's drainage system. It filters the blood and supports the immune system."

The pancreas, he explained, is a gland that sits deep in the abdomen and aids with digestion, among other things. Prednisone—which I had recently taken by the handful—I later learned is known to have an impact on the pancreas, affecting the secretions and, in high doses, causing damage to the organ itself.

The EAV also showed a few points that were high: the gall bladder and kidney, both of which support digestion and filtration, were in the seventies.

Daniel reconfigured the EAV machine to show my response to fungus, parasites, bacteria and viruses. "Hmmm," he said, watching the needle bounce around each time. "Looks like a full house inside you."

He didn't look alarmed, more bemused. And for me, this felt like a life sentence had been reduced to a parking ticket. The real culprit could be fungi, parasites, bacteria and viruses? If they could arrive, they could also leave. Any and all of those sounded less permanent and more appealing than the mystery of multiple sclerosis.

"Likely the parasites are everywhere," Daniel said. "Most will be gone in a week. I suspect this could be Lyme disease however, which is a nasty parasite. It takes a bit longer."

We walked back to the front of his offices, where Daniel and Christopher conferred and started pulling items off the shelf to help me begin my recovery. They handed me a protein powder to make a smoothie each morning so I could start my day with energy. They gave me olive leaf extract, which has antibacterial, antiviral and anti-inflammatory properties, to dissolve in water. There was a little bottle of Lugol's solution, an iodine solution to combat iodine deficiency, and magnesium oil to massage into my feet three times a day.

"Magnesium is depleted under stress," Daniel said. "It helps with nerve transition and muscle strength. And the body absorbs it more efficiently through skin."

Daniel gave me liquid vitamin D3 and a detox remedy to help clean up my lymphatic system. And to help the body detox faster, he recommended I come back each day for "exercise with oxygen therapy," or EWOT, and to sit in the infrared sauna. For the EWOT, I could sit on the recumbent bike, read, put on a mask and inhale straight oxygen—which Daniel and Christopher said would help with nerve regeneration. And the sauna was to speed detoxification. Unlike a traditional sauna, an infrared one allows the body to get hotter without that uncomfortable feeling of your skin burning. Because I couldn't help myself, I asked a dozen questions about whether they would help me and what the potential side effects would be. Daniel answered them all to my satisfaction: it was clear my symptoms wouldn't get worse from these treatments, and they seemed innocuous enough. And the best-case scenario? The combination would catapult me back to perfect health. I made a series of appointments to bike and sit in the sauna, thanked Daniel and walked outside with Christopher.

Back at the apartment, I took out my notebook to jot down ideas from this meeting. It occurred to me that I felt like I was in good hands for the first time since this whole process began. Both Daniel and Christopher had shared loads of detailed information and had worked hard to make sure I understood. Equally important, these two men listened to me and patiently answered my questions, neither dismissing my concerns nor disregarding my fear. Maybe it's just a journalist's tendency, but I've long been skeptical when people give directions and then close the conversation. "Because I said so" never inspired much confidence in me. It was my body and my health we were discussing, and they seemed to believe, as I did, that I needed to take the lead role in caring for both.

As I reviewed my notes, their theories made sense to me. I was also glad their advice didn't come with pages of disclaimers about liver failure or suicidal tendencies as the pharmaceutical solutions did.

Christopher came by later with a big bag of tricks: vitamins B and E, flaxseed oil, *Gingko biloba* supplements, a multivitamin and digestive enzymes.

"We talked about getting rid of the viruses, bacteria and other garbage at Daniel's place," he said. "This is part of the nourish plan. You're starving yourself."

"What?" I interrupted. "I eat so healthy."

"No, it's not that," he said. "Most foods are grown far away, picked green and shipped around the world. When they arrive in the grocery, they've often lost most of their nutrients. That's why we need to supplement our food with vitamins."

This sounded reasonable and vitamins never hurt anyone, as far as I knew. For the next few days, I fell into an easy routine. I'd wake up in the morning, practice yoga and sit in meditation with the friendly, dancing Buddhas. Then I'd make a shake with fruit and vegan protein powder and take my remedies and supplements. I'd shower and head out the door and walk twenty-five minutes to Yaletown. I'd say hello to Daniel and pick something from his library.

On the bike with my oxygen mask, I read about brain health, liver function, vitamins and minerals. Every day, I'd ride and read, ride and read. Gathering information and actively withholding judgment, I felt like I was making progress. I was doing something on my own behalf.

After my ride and read session, I'd fill a pitcher of water and sit in the sauna for thirty minutes. Inside the heat, I watched sweat rolling down my arms and dripping down my legs, and I imagined all kinds of toxins draining out with each drop. During these times, I'd be reminded of how kind Bruce was being—especially since he couldn't be here yet—and I was again grateful.

Afterward, I'd shower, get dressed and find Christopher outside to go for lunch at some vegan, raw foods palace.

After a few days, I was so relaxed that my shoulders had dropped again to a new resting spot. I could let go of the tension in my neck and back because I was doing my part, and I had a team working with me to help me heal. I still had questions and concerns, only now I felt like I was on an adventure, a quest to get to the bottom of it, a journey with allies to find answers and resolve symptoms.

On day five of the Canadian adventure, Christopher picked me up in Yaletown and drove through Stanley Park across the bridge into West Vancouver. He had made an appointment with Dr. Mack Brown.

An older gentleman, Dr. Brown had been a family physician for decades. His small waiting room overflowed with characters of a standard family practice: a mother with her son, an older couple, a receptionist talking on the phone while simultaneously answering questions from people in the room. He had old magazines, a few new ones and books.

We waited ten minutes until Dr. Brown ushered us into his office. Comfy in my blue jeans and sweater, I lay down on a gray examination table with a camera overhead. As the mechanical arm moved the camera over me, Brown took an X-ray of my left hip and my lower spine. It took five minutes, and he reviewed the results with me immediately. No anxious waiting, no nasty phone call days later.

"Your spine is normal density for a woman your age, but your hip is a little low," Brown said. He showed me a small graph with a bright blue bar marking T-scores, or average bone densities in women as they age. Generally, women in their twenties have a T-score of around 0. In the midforties, the blue bar starts sloping down, and then evens out near –2.0 in the early sixties.

Above the blue bar was a dark green color and below it, bars of light green, yellow, orange and red. The dot representing my lumbar spine was in the healthy blue bar, although near the bottom of it. My T-score there was –0.5. The dot for the tip of my femur was below that in the light green. My T-score on that one was –1.4, which means low bone density. Less than –2.5 signals osteoporosis.

Brown asked about my exercise routine, how much physical activity I did and how much of it was weight bearing. I told him I'd been a runner for twenty-some years. I had run a handful of marathons and routinely ran 5Ks and 10Ks.

"Then you shouldn't be low. You should be above the normal range," he said. The reason for the discrepancy, he thought, was that

I wasn't absorbing calcium, and the most likely reason for that was a vitamin D deficiency.

"Oh, yeah, I have that," I said a little too enthusiastically. "That was the one test Silver agreed to do for me before I left Denver and the number was twelve. I guess normal is between thirty and one hundred parts per something or other."

I had sent all my test results to Christopher, who flipped through the pile of pages he was carrying and handed the vitamin D page to the doctor. "Oh shoot," Brown said. He knew the test I'd taken and that vitamin D gets involved in almost every bodily function: it's critical for bone health, cell growth, nerve and muscular strength, immune function and mood stabilization.

"I know," Christopher said. "When I saw that, I wondered how she could even walk across the floor."

Brown scanned the page and turned around to get a pill bottle off his desk. He filled it with ten 1-milligram doses of vitamin D, or ten pills with 50,000 international units (IUs). "Take these for ten days, then go to ten thousand IU a day," he said. The Recommended Daily Intake (RDI) for women my age is 15 micrograms, or 600 IU a day. Brown acknowledged that some people thought 50,000 IU was too much, that it could lead to vitamin D toxicity. He disagreed based on common sense—in direct sunlight, the human body produces 20,000 IU in about twenty minutes—and his own experience.

"I stumbled onto vitamin D about six years ago," he said. "I was breaking too many bones."

At the time, Brown had a bone-density scan done and found himself in the orange osteoporosis bar at the bottom of the graph. He started himself on high doses of vitamin D and stuck with it. He stopped breaking bones and had himself scanned again a few years later, and saw a remarkable difference. Now his bone density was higher than expected for men his age. And, he said, taking the vitamin D improved his health in general. He felt better and had more energy.

We talked a few more minutes about vitamin D, and I began to feel like he was another expert I could trust, another guy on the team I was assembling who wanted to help. I was feeling so confident and comfortable that I thought that maybe, just maybe, I could ask the really scary question without bursting into tears or flames or anything else.

I took a deep breath and asked about MS. "I'm really scared," I said. "I don't think that's what I have, but the MRI showed lesions, and the doctor in Denver seemed so sure."

Brown looked at me, kindly and gently, with empathy and patience.

In a small voice that barely traveled across the silence, I said, "Do you think I can heal?"

"Oh shit," he said, like an old cowboy. "I'm so radical, I think everything can heal."

Right then and there, I decided I loved him. I thought about kissing him and decided against it. Instead, I thanked him profusely, took his card in case I had questions and thanked him again.

*I'm so radical, I think everything can heal.* I must have repeated the line a hundred times that night. I thought about Brown saying that and I thought about Lance Armstrong. Seemingly a hundred years ago, in my sportswriter life, Nike had invited me and a dozen other journalists to visit its campus in Oregon and spend time getting to know its cycling gear. In other words, Nike loaded us up with shoes, shorts and jerseys and loaned us bikes for a couple of days to test drive.

To sweeten the deal, Nike brought in its biggest cycling celebrity, although he wasn't that big outside of cycling at the time. This was a few years before Lance had won any Tours de France, so he was just a cocky Texan who rode by us one day on the road. At night, we all went to dinner. The Nike PR staff sat with the journalists, and Lance sat with his girlfriend at another table. Since we were all in the same restaurant, this counted as our dinner with Lance. A week later, he was diagnosed with testicular cancer that had spread through his brain and lungs. Doctors told him it was over. His coach later told me, "He was circling the drain. Doctors told him to get his affairs in order."

I don't know what Lance said to that, but in my imagination, when the doctors told him he was going to die, he responded, "Yeah, thanks. I've got other plans. I've got a few Tours de France to win." Then he pulled himself together, found the treatment that worked for him and got on with life.

As I thought about Lance and heard Brown saying, "I'm so radical, I think everything can heal," I wished I could rewrite history so that I too could have said something defiant in the moment of diagnosis. Silver would say, "You have MS," and I would say, "Yeah, thanks. I've got other plans."

No matter, I was making other plans anyway.

CHAPTER 7

# THE TRAUMA OF IT ALL

I have explored every city I've lived in by foot. Even Los Angeles I learned by walking and running. I'd never lived in Vancouver, but after a week with an apartment, a project and a routine, I wanted to remedy that mistake. I geared up in running clothes and my beloved Brooks Adrenalines. I'd been running in this same brand of shoes for five years, buying a new pair every four or five months when the old ones went flat. The shoes were as familiar as any item I'd ever worn. I'd run in them in hot weather and cold, slush and sand, on three-hour slogs and ten-minute mind-clearing jogs.

Three months, however, had gone by since my last run. There were reasons, of course: brutally cold days in Denver, the MRI, the diagnosis, and then the crazy-making steroids that wreaked havoc on my health. My feet still felt a little awkward. There was no tingling, but something was tweaking the nerve between my toes, giving me that weird flip-flop feeling still. But I felt so inspired by my meetings with Daniel and Brown, and I had stopped taking the steroids, so I decided it was time to hit the pavement again. Perhaps by now, the steroids were fully out of my system because I discovered I could notice the feeling in my feet without obsessing over it.

I laced up and headed out the door and down the block into Stanley Park, which rivals New York's Central Park in terms of beauty—and it may win, because it has more hills and water on all sides.

As I cruised along, hearing the familiar and hypnotic one-two beat, I looked at the harbor on one side and the dense trees on the other and thought how glad I was that I'd come. Even without Bruce, Vancouver felt like a warm hug. I was eating healthy food, inhaling crisp and clean air, and stuffing my brain with liberating concepts.

The next day I woke with the familiar feeling in my quads, that slight touch of discomfort that's only physical. Mentally, that little burn was as comforting and reassuring as sunlight after a storm. That subtle stiffness told me my body had been working and that I'd endured and overcome the combination of pavement, lactic acid and an hour of elevated heart rate. The feeling was an old friend saying I was stronger today than I had been yesterday.

I finished my morning routine and met Christopher in Yaletown just before lunch. He had one more doctor for me to meet, Guillaume Martin, a charming and good-looking Frenchman with dark, dark hair and dark, dark eyes and an office full of photos of stealth bombers and jets flying in formation. On each of his shelves, model airplanes stood ready to take off.

"I've got a thing for planes too," I said. "I learned to fly Cessnas when I was in college. And I got to fly in an F-18 with the Blue Angels."

His eyes lit up. "Really?" he said, sounding more like a little kid than a respected doctor with spacious offices in a sophisticated city.

"Someone from the team called the paper I was working for and offered to take a journalist for a ride. My editor knew I'd do it in a heartbeat."

"I would have done it too," Dr. Martin said. "I was a flight surgeon for the French Air Force."

He pointed to the planes on his wall and told me how he got to ride with the great athletes who piloted them and how working with the air force spurred his interest in human performance. The pilots who flew those jets competed at the highest levels of human capability; their reactions were instantaneous and precise, their vision clear and their nervous systems calm in the most harried of situations. As Dr. Martin got to know the pilots, he wondered if everyone couldn't go through life with the same poise and perfection, if they received the proper training and education.

Intrigued by this idea, Dr. Martin studied neurophysiology, human performance and the barriers to peak performance. Since trauma ranks among the biggest barriers to performance, he studied its impacts on the nervous system. And the more he learned, the more he wanted to know. He wanted to measure the impacts of physical, cognitive and emotional trauma to see if the impacts of all three were reversible.

Dr. Martin's curiosity led him to accumulate degrees, diplomas and accolades from Western medical institutions. In addition, he studied Eastern healing traditions, including acupuncture. In creating his practice, he worked to provide a drugless, noninvasive and holistic approach to healing.

Drugless? Noninvasive? Holistic? Given my aversion even to Tylenol (let alone those awful steroids), Dr. Martin and his team sounded like my kind of people. They worked to get rid of symptoms and restore function by understanding how the brain responded to incidents in life. Instead of viewing each symptom as a separate event with a separate treatment, they explored and considered whether one problem could create multiple symptoms or whether many issues could contribute to one symptom. In either event, they looked to remove the cause of the symptom instead of merely masking the symptom itself.

I liked what he said and the way he spoke. To me, the human body seemed too complicated and too interconnected for the restricted, linear logic I felt Silver was selling: tingling plus lesions equals MS, and if it's MS, then take drugs. And Dr. Martin, it seemed, agreed with me. He told me to call him Guy, which rhymed with *tea*, and said he'd like to interview me before a physical exam. For ninety minutes, he asked about all aspects of my life. We both took notes as he asked about falls, illnesses, broken bones and surgeries—anything that could have contributed to the tingling or the lesions. He asked if I could recall hitting my head or tumbling off a bike.

"Sure," I said. "I'm not a particularly good athlete, but I don't let that stop me. I went over the handle bars on a bike about ten years ago, and I fell off a horse or two, years before that."

"And tell him about the time you were hypoxic," Christopher added.

The day before, I had told Christopher about a trip to Ecuador where a brilliant photographer named Tony DiZinno saved my life. On assignment for *ESPN* magazine, Tony and I were assigned to shoot and write about an epic adventure race in which teams of four hiked, mountain biked, kayaked and climbed their way through a 250-mile unmarked course in the Andes. They had to reach thirty checkpoints along the way using a compass and topo map. Early in the race, one checkpoint was the summit of Cotopaxi, a 19,347-foot volcano.

In the quest for a great magazine story, Tony and I chased the teams to the base of the volcano and started slogging our way to the warming hut at seventeen thousand feet. At eleven o'clock at night, it was below freezing and snow was falling. Tony seemed to be moving much more quickly than I was. So I sat down.

Tony turned to me and said, "What are you doing?"

"You're moving so much faster, I don't want to hold you up."

"So, what are you doing?"

"I'm just going to wait here," I said.

"Wait for what?"

"Daylight."

It made perfect sense to me and zero sense to Tony. He connected my backpack to his on a short rope and hauled my ass to the warming hut. It was no more than five minutes up the trail but, loopy as I was in the elevated air, I would have sat in the snow all by myself all night long just five minutes from safety. Inside the hut, Tony found hot cider for me to drink, gave me a sleeping bag to wrap up in, and rubbed my hands and feet while asking questions to check my sanity. Somehow, it returned.

Still, Tony was taking no chances. In the early morning, around three, when teams were gearing up to leave for the summit, Tony told me I was going nowhere and assigned someone else to look after me while he hiked up and shot some of the most beautiful images I've ever seen.

I told Guy this story in case it somehow had contributed to my health issues. He nodded and jotted it down.

The conversation went on, covering the greatest hits in the Jody calamity file—the time I fell off a rock while bouldering; the time I got clobbered by a runaway windsurfer; the time I tried windsurfing myself and banged into the mast. We covered the extensive orthodontia I had as a teenager and the crazy anti-pigeon-toe thing my mother had me wear as a toddler. I told stories that I had never told—not even to myself because they had seemed inconsequential and unconnected—or embarrassing. But as I told and told, no one looked surprised, and Guy took notes.

When he'd concluded the interview and we were ready for the physical exam, we went into another room where the walls, floor and ceiling were painted black. Barefoot, I stood on a platform on one side of the room, where white spots on the walls allowed Guy to measure my height, the height of each shoulder and how everything lined up from the side view. The wall directly across from me had a series of white dots in a cross, like the center of a riflescope.

The platform itself measured balance, wobbliness and pressure under my feet. I stood as still as I could with my eyes shut, and then with them open, while Guy wrote down the measurements. Good balance, he explained, shows that information is running smoothly through the nervous system from the feet to the brain, and from brain to feet. Essentially, if I had good balance, it was unlikely I had MS.

After a few more balance drills, Guy stood before me and had me follow a pen in his hand with my eyes only. Then, the same drill with one eye covered and then the other. Finally, he had me cover one eye as he moved the pen up and down and asked me to identify, looking through the tip of the pen, which spot I saw on the wall. I wanted to get it right and knew that was impossible. No right answers. No wrong ones. I just told him what I saw.

Guy was kind, relaxed and more than a little sexy. And I felt like we were in this together. If all doctor's appointments were this encouraging and entertaining, I'd go more often—I was sure of it.

When the exam was over, I put my shoes on and we went back to the conference room. Guy told me my static posture could be improved with therapy. And that my balance was good but could also be improved. This was a relief, because in my mind, anything that could get better couldn't be part of a permanent degenerative disease.

"I noticed," he said, "as we continued the drills and your eyes became tired, there was some hesitation, some fluctuation between the left and right eyes. It was as if your brain couldn't decide which side was dominant."

He looked at my hands, which were on the table. "Are you right or left handed?"

"Right," I said, looking at my hands to see what he was seeing.

"Yet you wear your watch on the right wrist."

"Yeah, when I started wearing a watch, no one told me not to wear it on the right, so I did and got used to it. If I need to write something, you know with a pen," I said, scribbling an imaginary signature, "I take it off and put it on the table."

"I think you were left handed, or ambidextrous, and you trained yourself to be right handed," Guy said. "And that causes a little confusion or hesitation between the hemispheres of your brain." The brain and body, he said, work more efficiently if we work with their natural tendencies.

Guy and I talked a little longer and I asked him about the lesions—braver now since Brown said everything could heal. Guy said he'd look at the MRI, so I gave him the CD with the images that the hospital had sent me in Denver, thanked him and said good-bye.

That night, I had dinner in the neighborhood with a friend named Nikki. It was great to spend time with her, this friend from another part of my life—we'd met at surf camp in Costa Rica—and to talk about politics and surfing and men. Then, of course, the conversation turned to health, and I'd forgotten that Nikki had once done some sleuthing for her own health. She'd been feeling fatigued and achy and went through a few frustrating rounds with physicians.

Each had different ideas and none could help. Finally a naturopath helped her determine that wheat was causing the problems. She changed her diet and life improved.

"I guess grains aren't always part of a healthy diet," I said.

"They aren't for me," Nikki said. "And I swear by my naturopath. Here's her card."

If I really lived in Vancouver, instead of just "borrowing" it as my city for a few weeks, I'd have made an appointment immediately. Absolutely, I would have. Instead, I stayed on the Christopher plan until I went home.

The next morning, I went through my usual routine: stretch, meditate, protein shake, twenty-five minute walk to Yaletown for a bit on the bike and time in the sauna. Christopher picked me up from Daniel's office, and as we were driving to lunch, he told me he was going to meet with Guy that afternoon and he'd let me know what they recommended.

"You're going to do *what*?" I said. "The two of you are going to get together and talk about me…without me? No, if there's going to be a meeting about my health, I should be there."

Christopher looked hurt and stunned—and truth be told, I was nearly as surprised by my outburst. Christopher had been nothing but nice to me and had done nothing but share his experience and hard-earned wisdom. Same for Guy. And yet I was afraid they were going to talk about me behind closed doors, then come out and tell me what to do. Weren't we supposed to be a team here, working together to help me get better?

"Did you speak to Bruce too?" I asked.

"He wanted to know how you were doing," Christopher said, thinking he'd been helpful and looking confused.

I sighed. "Look, if we're a team working on my health, I really have to understand all the decisions. Giving up control is still too scary."

Bruce, Christopher and Guy had been incredibly kind and taken a lot of time to try to help me get to the root of this issue. But my earlier experiences still haunted me.

"Look, I'd like to take that appointment. He was going to tell me what he saw in my MRI and if he can recommend a treatment. If you need to talk to him about other things, can you do it another time?"

Christopher looked braced for battle and then relaxed. "OK, fine," he said, as if it wasn't worth the fight. We drove on in silence.

When I walked into Guy's office, he led me into the conference room and took a seat opposite me. "I looked at your MRIs," he said, "and they are very good pictures, very clear. The lesions are certainly there, and yes, it could be MS, but it could also be many other things. Trauma could explain the lesions, or they could come from vascular issues, a lack of oxygen to the tissue, for example."

There was a range of other explanations, he said, adding that illness is a degenerative process, worsening over time.

"Trauma may lead to illness but it doesn't have to," Guy said.

"I'm not sure I understand."

"Traumatic events could trigger a downward slide into a long-term illness but they don't have to," he said. "Judging from the exam, your history, the MRI and how you move, I'd say you are more trauma than illness. You are not ill, and this is a good thing."

For the second time in one week, I wanted to kiss the doctor and stopped myself. *I am not ill? Wahoo!* This was not only a good thing. It was a very, very good thing, an excellent thing, among the greatest things I'd ever heard, right up there with "everything can heal."

"Even better," Guy said, "the effects of trauma can be reversed."

A wave of energy, a warm surge of power, came up from my belly into my chest and filled me with joy. *The effects can be reversed? Where I do I sign up? I am ready, let's reverse this weird ride. Let's get going* now.

"Great," I said. "How do we do it? When can we start?"

Guy smiled and his eyes softened as if to say, "Hold it there, tiger."

"This is not an overnight process," he said. "You spent years accumulating the trauma and the effects. We'd have to do more extensive testing to design a program for you. Typically, my clients work with me for three months. They come in two or three times a week for a combination of acupuncture, nutritional coaching, exercises and other therapies, depending on their needs. This is a very specific, individualized treatment plan."

*Three* months? I'd have loved to stay, but I had a house, work, a dog and a life in Denver. "I'd have to move here for three months?"

"Not necessarily; I work with out-of-town patients. They typically come one week a month and we do a number of treatments the week they're here."

*Hmm*. That sounded possible, though expensive. "How effective is it?"

He said he'd worked with similar patients in the past and that since he opened the clinic in 1997, for all patients with a range of mysterious symptoms, he'd had an 85 percent success rate.

I liked those odds. "What would it cost?"

"Depends on the treatment program and the number of different therapies," Guy said. "Three months usually costs around fifteen thousand dollars."

That was the sum total in my bank account. But then again, this was my health and I was tired of tingling. Plus, I would have paid anything to know for sure it wasn't the sign of a chronic, often painful, potentially fatal condition. And he was saying, for $15,000, we could solve the problem, not just mask it. We *could* reverse the effects of this trauma. Mentally, I did a quick calculation to compare his plan with Silver's. The former was noninvasive and drugless, with an 85 percent chance of success for a cool $15,000. The latter included routine injections of a toxic substance that didn't even attempt to solve the problem. Not permanently. At best, interferons (the likely treatment I'd have to go with) merely slowed the descent into hell in about one-third of the people who tried them. And they cost $3,000 a month for life, which for me, could be a while. All my grandparents had lived into their nineties. Three grand a month, twelve months a year, forty-five years—that's $1.6 million with no guarantees.

As I did the math, I forgot completely about all the other data I had been accumulating. I didn't compare Guy's or Silver's options to what Daniel and Dr. Brown had been telling me earlier: that basically, I was fine; I just needed to change my diet, do a few other things and take vitamins. That all sounded great, but despite second-guessing Silver, I had bought into his idea that I had a great big problem and needed a great, big solution, like Guy's.

I even forgot what Christopher had said before: that most people want to be told what to do. I apparently wanted a neurologist to tell me what to do—I just didn't want it to be Silver or for the directions to include drugs. To me, fifteen grand and time with this French doc seemed a far better option.

But I wasn't quite ready to commit. So I told Guy I'd figure out if I could spend time in Vancouver and be in touch.

That night, Bruce arrived from Mexico. I was eager to see him and tell him the latest, and ecstatic to see how excited he was to see me too. We met on a street corner and before I stepped onto the curb, he picked me up with a bear hug and then held my hand as we walked along the waterfront. When the dusk became darker, we went for a drink, then dinner, and another drink. He came back to the apartment, and we shared an exciting and sleepless night together. The next morning, he caught a cab to an early business meeting, and after a few hours, Terry came to give me a ride to the airport. A brief but beautiful visit.

On the flight, I sat by the window and watched the scenery for three hours and 1,400 miles. The sun was out, everything looked clean and new, and my attitude was infinitely better returning to Denver than it had been when I left.

I landed overflowing with ideas. Could whatever's going on with me be attributed to a vitamin deficiency? A heavy metal toxicity? Lyme disease? Trauma? An alignment issue? Or anything that could be reversed? I was certain that one of those things was the real issue and that my immune system was *not* attacking me, only doing what it was supposed to do—clearing away bugs and head colds and everything else the environment could toss at me.

Hope, optimism and questions spilled out of my pores. In Vancouver, I had learned a new model of working *with* doctors, of teaming with them to move me toward health. I liked feeling that I was part of a problem-solving crew, and I felt confident that a variety of expert opinions could zero in on the solution more quickly and more completely than anyone alone.

However, while I loved my team in Vancouver, they were still in Vancouver, which would make it expensive and difficult for me to coordinate my care. I figured Silver was my doctor in Denver and together we could recruit other experts also covered by my insurance and re-create something similar here. Why not? We both wanted me to heal, didn't we?

I called his office. He had said, "If you have questions, call me. I will call you back within twenty-four hours." I was eager to reach a solution, and although we hadn't known each other long, he knew more about my health than any other doctor in Denver.

No response.

So I waited twenty-four hours and called again. Nothing. I called the day after that and still nothing. But I still thought he could help so I called every day for two weeks and received no response.

I was confused. I understood that he was a busy man, but a promise was still a promise. Plus, Silver had seemed so eager to call me at home and deliver the diagnosis, had even volunteered to stay late that day to explain the bad news. But now that I had questions and thought I could heal, he was nowhere to be found?

It didn't make sense to me, and I really wanted an answer, or at least some kind of closure from him, so I kept dialing. At the end of the second week of daily calls, I resorted to one of my least favorite tactics I learned as a reporter. I never liked doing it, and yet sometimes "phone banking" was the only option. I called Silver every hour starting at nine in the morning. I called at nine, at ten, at eleven, and on and on, until three in the afternoon. When I'd talked to the same nurse eight times, I asked her if it was making any difference.

"Is he getting these messages, and is he any more likely to call me back? Or am I just making your life miserable?"

"Well," she said, "he knows you've been calling."

# CHAPTER 8

# LARGER IDEAS AND LESSER EVILS

With Silver out of the picture, I needed to find new options. I wanted people with big ideas and a holistic view of health. I also wanted smart people, so I went to the one place I always find a collection of them: the library.

The downtown Denver Public Library looks to me from the outside like a box of crayons. And the light inside feels like the daylight outside. I walked deep into the stacks to find books on doctors, health and healing. Quickly, I discovered Dr. Andrew Weil, a medical doctor, naturopath and founder of the Institute for Integrative Medicine at the University of Arizona. A prolific author, he wrote *Health and Healing* in 1983. It was easy to read and made sense to me. I skimmed some of his other works too and liked the way he described integrative medicine as a "healing-oriented medicine that takes account of the whole person (body, mind, and spirit), including all aspects of lifestyle. It emphasizes the therapeutic relationship and makes use of all appropriate therapies, both conventional and alternative."

Sounded like the comprehensive approach I wanted, so I used the library's computer to find local doctors who had trained with Weil.

I found Maureen Duncan, who had a picture of herself with Weil and a mission statement on her website. She said she believed in the body's natural healing abilities and would work to facilitate that process. As an extension of the Hippocratic oath, and its directive to "do no harm," she wrote that she always started with the least invasive and least toxic treatments and therapies first.

Now that sounds more like it. I called and made an appointment.

Dr. Duncan had long blond hair and wore little or no makeup. She looked to be in her late forties. She seemed like a mom—not my mom, but someone's mom—in that she seemed efficient and caring and capable. Her office was big and open, with an exam table near the window, a desk with chairs on both sides, and bookcases filled with titles like *Our Bodies, Ourselves*; *Perfect Healing*; and *The Vitamin D Cure*. She interviewed me for an hour or more, listening, taking notes and asking follow-up questions. I was relaxing a bit and thinking that maybe this was the norm and that the "wham-bam-thank-you-ma'am" folks at my HMO were the aberration.

Duncan looked in my ears, my nose and my eyes. She tested my reflexes, felt the glands in my neck and felt my abdomen. "That doesn't feel so good. Is it always that hard? Do you feel bloated after you eat?"

I didn't know. I rarely thought about my belly.

After the physical exam, Dr. Duncan moved back to her desk and I took a seat across from her. She said that she had several patients with MS and that I didn't move like they did. She believed there could be other explanations for the tingling, which had shrunk to that flip-flop feeling between my toes. She suggested several tests, including a full thyroid panel, a nutrient analysis and a test for heavy metal toxicity.

"And you should journal about MS and what it means to you," she said. "I have patients who have it, and it's not that big a deal to them. You seem really upset by it, so journaling will help you to figure out why it's so upsetting to you."

Sounded like a good idea.

"Also," she asked, "do you have a will? You should have a will."

*Um, no.*

Until that last question, I was feeling confident. But I shook off the sinking feeling and made an appointment to return for the nutrient and heavy metal tests, which I'd pay for out of pocket, the same as I'd pay for my time with her. With my insurance, I had to pay if I wanted to see anyone out of network, and the network didn't include doctors like Duncan, who spent hours with a patient. Still, for the thyroid panel, a fairly conventional test, I figured I could find some way to use my insurance.

Duncan thought I could too, so she wrote down the requested test on her prescription pad. I drove from her office to the HMO's main hospital ten minutes away. I took the page to the lab and dropped my insurance ID card into the cue on the lab technician's desk. When the woman called my name, I approached the counter.

"Oh, no, no, no, this has to come from a network doctor or you'll pay out of pocket."

I asked what it would cost, and she didn't know. She looked shocked, as if I was the first person to request a full thyroid panel. And the first to ask what it cost.

"Well, you could get the test and when you get your bill, you'll see what it costs," she said smiling and not joking.

I took the page from Duncan's pad and walked outside, cursing the system. Simultaneously, I started planning another way to use the system. If I had to get a network doc to prescribe a thyroid panel, fine. I called to make an appointment with Dr. Wise, the curly-haired doctor who sent me to Silver.

The next afternoon, I found myself in the now-familiar waiting room until a nurse came to walk me to an exam room, where I could wait some more.

Just glancing around the room made me a little queasy. Bad memories and all. I started thinking I was sick. Why else would I be in this room? I went through my evidence: a few doctors had said not MS. I was symptom-free without using the MS drugs. No more tingling, no weakness, no numbness, no vision issues. No nothing except for the phantom flip-flop feeling in my toes, but that didn't bother me so much since I had mentioned it to my friend Lisa. "That's so cool," she said. "It's always summer inside your shoes."

I sat on the examination table flipping through magazines, waiting for Dr. Wise and wondering if trying to use my insurance was worth it. Just being in the cold room, alone with paper crinkling on the table under my legs, made me nervous. I looked at my watch—it'd been twenty minutes since I had been brought in and thirty minutes since I'd first arrived—and heard the door open.

Dr. Wise looked the same as the last time I'd seen her: dry, curly black hair framed her narrow face, and pale skin stretched tense over her nose. She had thin forearms and was almost birdlike in appearance, a little like my mom.

"What's up?" she asked.

"I'd like to get a thyroid panel," I said.

"Why?" she asked.

"I'm seeing another doctor for a second opinion, and she thinks it's a good idea."

Without looking at me, Dr. Wise sat at the desk and opened my electronic file on the computer.

"Oh, you have MS," she said, off-handedly.

"I don't think so. That's what Dr. Silver thinks, but I've been seeking other opinions from other doctors, and based on the evidence, they don't believe I have MS."

Her posture changed. I watched her spine grow more rigid, her shoulders stiffen. And as she grew taller in her chair, I started to slump.

Without turning away from the computer, she twisted her head over her shoulder to look at me. I felt like she was trying to remember who I was. And jogging her memory seemed important.

"I came to see you when I had tingling in my fingers, and you sent me to see Dr. Silver. He ordered an MRI and called to tell me I had MS," I said.

Wise was still staring over her shoulder without saying anything. I couldn't see any recognition in her eyes, no sign that my words were landing, so I continued. "It's been a nightmare. I wish I never said anything about the tingling."

Now, the room—and her over-the-shoulder, birdlike gaze—felt oppressive, and I was becoming scared again. I could feel my shoulders rounding forward and my heart picking up speed.

Wise turned away again to look at the screen. "Did he discuss treatment options?"

Didn't matter what I had said, she was sticking to her talking points. "How are you going to treat it?" implies, without a doubt, that "it" exists.

I wasn't sure if I should repeat myself about seeking second opinions, so there was a brief silence.

To fill it, Wise repeated herself, "Did he discuss treatment options?"

Sometimes it's just easier to cave. "Yeah," I said. "He gave me four one-pagers, and they all look awful."

Dr. Wise swung around to face me and suddenly looked an awful lot like my mom. Specifically, she made the face my mom made to tell me I was ungrateful for something.

"For years," Dr. Wise said, "MS patients were dying for those drugs."

She narrowed her gaze and her nostrils flared as if to drive home the point. "They had no hope, and they were dying for those drugs."

I didn't want to die. Not for drugs. Not for anything. Not yet.

"Well, I'm not convinced I have MS, so I'm not thinking about the interferons right now."

"Well, I don't know what else could cause these lesions," she said, closing the computer file. Before I could say anything, she stood and left the room.

I don't think she'd seen the MRI—although I didn't get to ask her—so I didn't know if she was making assumptions about lesions she had never seen.

The conversation didn't seem finished though—she hadn't answered my question about ordering a thyroid test—so I assumed she was coming back.

Sitting on the examining table with my feet dangling over the edge, I was grateful that another doctor—one who *had* read the MRI, Dr. Martin—had other ideas. And, I thought, if Wise doesn't know what else could cause lesions, maybe she could talk to him or someone else with more information. Either way, for me, one doctor's ignorance was no reason to take drugs. I sat swinging my feet off the table and listening to the paper crinkle beneath my thighs when a nurse came in and looked startled to see me.

"What are you doing here?"

"Waiting for Dr. Wise to come back."

"She's not coming back. Is there something you need?"

*Compassion would be nice*, I thought. *I'd settle for a bit of kindness.*

I would have asked the nurse to order the test if I thought she could have. I left the hospital and paid out of pocket for the thyroid test and had results sent to Dr. Duncan.

When I went back to see her to review the results of all the tests, she said my thyroid numbers were well within the normal range.

The vitamin and nutrient panel was more interesting. I had plenty of B vitamins and not nearly enough D—which was surprising because I'd been basically mainlining both of them for nearly a month now. In antioxidants, I was low on vitamin E and coenzyme Q-10.

She handed me a stapled set of pages with results from the heavy metal test and as I read through, I saw the range for healthy populations were marked on the bar graph in yellow. The danger zone was, naturally, in red. With lead, I was far in the red, with more than double the acceptable range. On mercury, I had more than seventeen times the range. I kept reading down the list—OK on antimony, whatever that is; fine on barium; no problem on cadmium.

"What the hell is gadolinium?" I asked before I had time to think.

"That's the contrasting agent they use for MRIs," Duncan said.

The reference range for healthy people is less than 0.019 micrograms per gram. I had 2.918 micrograms, 153 times the normal amount.

"If heavy metals cause nerve damage, why would they inject that, knowing from the tingling that something was going on with my nerves?"

"C'mon," Duncan said. "What if it had revealed a tumor or something else that was causing your symptoms? You'd have wanted to know about it."

"I guess so. Still, no one told me it would stay in my body. No one even told me it was a heavy metal or what the contrasting agent was."

Duncan reassured me that we could remove all the metals with chelation. Since the body tucks metals into faraway corners, they are harder to remove than the lesser toxins we eliminate in the usual ways. To excrete the metals, a person has to ingest something that will bind to the metal and pull it out of the system. Cilantro and some algae are natural chelating agents, and there are chemical compounds that do the same job.

Duncan said heavy metal toxicity could explain the tingling. It sounded more logical than Silver's theory of the return-of-the-chicken-pox antibodies. It fit with what I'd learned in Canada. And, for sure, heavy metals didn't belong in my body. Removing them seemed like a reasonable idea.

She explained that chelation could take a while; she had done it herself and said it was worth it. She suggested I come to her office once a month so her nurse could give me an IV of the chelating agent, and three days of each week, I'd take four Chelex pills, which had natural and chemical chelating agents.

"Don't eat any seafood for twenty-four hours before the IV, and don't take your supplements on the days you take the Chelex—it will just take them all out anyway so it's a waste," she said.

Duncan also suggested I stop eating all gluten, the protein found in many grains, and all dairy products for one month.

I didn't ask too many questions but agreed to do it all: eliminate my soothing breads and pastas, get a monthly IV, swallow Chelex pills three days a week and nutritional supplements the other four. While the plan sounded awful in some ways, it seemed infinitely better than the one alternative that still sat heavy at the center of my focus: MS and injections for the rest of my life. And this plan didn't sound too tricky. I could always tell what food contained gluten and dairy, right? *Ingredients are obvious.* Or so I thought.

CHAPTER 9

# FAMILY TIES

"How ya doing, Jo?"

My dad calls me Jo most of the time. Sometimes he calls me Curly and occasionally Shorty. My sister and I are just one year apart, and when we were kids, he'd look at us and say, "Now which one of you is Shorty and which one is Curly?"

I'm not sure what he calls Ellen these days. Mostly, I'm Jo.

"Pretty good, Dad," I said.

He asked what the new doctor had to say, and I told him about the chelation and that she suggested I give up gluten and dairy. I said I was going to, as if it were no big deal, as if I hadn't started so many days for so many years with a bagel and cream cheese and finished with pasta and Parmesan cheese.

"I wouldn't change my diet for any doctor," my dad said. And it's true. Doctors must have told him to give up desserts and eat more vegetables until they were blue in the face. It's got to be a standard part of the diabetes rap. And yet, ten years after his diagnosis, my father would rather adjust medications than alter his diet.

I told myself I didn't feel that strongly about food. I liked it, liked eating out, even liked cooking it—I just liked my health more.

Food seemed an easy thing to change, and not for any doctor. I was taking vitamins and chelating agents, and avoiding gluten and dairy for me. Just for me.

Or so I thought. But who knows? Maybe Christopher was right when he said, "Most people do as they're told." Maybe I was no different, and my dad was.

"So, let's pick a weekend and meet in New York," he said.

Once a year, he and I would meet in Manhattan, catch a play and try a new restaurant or go back to old favorites. After a few days, we'd take the train to the suburbs to see my cousins.

We picked a weekend and decided to reverse the order. We each flew into LaGuardia and made our way to Grand Central to catch a train out of the city. In a leafy green town up the Hudson River, we went to a neighborhood Italian restaurant with my cousin Dawn, her partner Jon and their newly adopted son, Andrei, who had spent the first four years of his life in an orphanage in Russia. No matter, he looked surprisingly like his mom. He and Dawn both had light coloring, dark eyes and round, happy cheeks.

Someone ordered fried calamari and mozzarella sticks for the table, and I watched as everyone else enjoyed them. For dinner, I ate a simple fish dish with rice and drank a glass of wine. My father ordered a frozen strawberry daiquiri and zoned out as Dawn tried to keep the adult conversation going while teaching Andrei restaurant etiquette.

"It's good to stay in your chair while eating," she said gently, like a patient kindergarten teacher. "Remember? We talked about this."

For his part, Andrei seemed happy to stay seated and eat, until eventually he grew bored. From his chair, he started flirting with a girl at the next table. She looked his age and was adopted too, from China. Andrei charmed her for a while and then moved on to flirt with both her parents.

"It's amazing," I said. "He's only been here, what? Two years? And look at him go. He has such a big vocabulary and no accent."

"It hasn't even been a year," Jon said, "Dawn has done so much work with him. She worked on language and physical stuff too. When he got here, he couldn't do anything across the midline."

Jon reached his right hand across his body to the left, then the left hand to the right to show me what he meant. "He couldn't even crawl, and his balance was awful," he said. "He'd spent most of his time in the orphanage in a high chair, strapped in. He didn't get to do normal kid stuff."

Adoption can be painfully slow, and many times the kids arrive with special challenges. As a child psychologist who teaches developmentally disabled children, Dawn was probably better equipped than most to handle the wait and help a child overcome obstacles. And she was determined to do both. She worked with the adoption agency for years before she and Jon were able to bring Andrei home on a long flight from Moscow.

Dawn and Jon lived in a light- and plant-filled home on a hilly acre and a half. My father and I stayed overnight, and in the morning, Jon gave me a tour of the property, which was covered with trees, roots, rocks, fallen leaves, bushes and random holes here and there—it all sloped down to a creek. Beautiful, their yard seemed perfect for a kid with an imagination. As Jon and I talked, Andrei ran all over the place. Just three feet tall, give or take, he vaulted himself over logs, shimmied between branches and stopped suddenly to bend to the dirt and examine a bug or something creepy and crawly on the ground. Just as suddenly, he'd pop back up and sprint toward us.

Later, inside the house, I said to Dawn, "He's doing great."

"Yeah, he's so amazing," she said. "When I took him to preschool, they wanted to put him in the class with the developmentally disabled kids. I said no. I didn't want my kid to be the highest achieving kid in the room."

Dawn enrolled him in a private school part-time, and while taking a long maternity leave, she played with him every day, ran drills and designed games to help develop his coordination, language and confidence. When she took him back to the same school district six months later to talk about options for kindergarten, they decided they must have been mistaken; he wasn't disabled after all and could enroll in the regular kindergarten class.

*Developmental disabilities can last forever, but forever's a funny thing,* I thought, remembering what Christopher had told me: "The only thing they know for certain is that it's forever. If they diagnosis MS and it goes away, then it must have been a misdiagnosis. It's bullshit."

Dawn and I were standing in the kitchen watching Andrei out the window. "I'm so proud of him," she said.

"I'm so proud of you," I said. And I meant it. She was ridiculously inspiring to me. Andrei came with a label, a diagnosis that promised to limit his future. Dawn ignored it and proved that, with compassion, persistence and training, anything was possible.

As my father and I rode the train to Manhattan the next day, we couldn't stop talking about Andrei.

"He's a cute little guy, isn't he?" my dad said. "And his vocabulary is amazing."

"I know," I said. "Dawn and Jon—wow, it's just really good parenting. It's great to watch them with him."

The train rolled into Manhattan, and as we stepped into Grand Central Station, I felt the familiar surge of energy and anxiety. All those people moving with aggression, determination and indifference made me uneasy. When I lived in New York, I avoided Times Square at all costs and mostly went out on weeknights rather than brave the torrents of people rushing in for a Saturday night in Manhattan. "Weekends are for amateurs," a friend of mine always said, and, some days, I agreed. Other days, I knew I was the amateur who couldn't play with the pros.

My dad, on the other hand, grew up in New York—on the Grand Concourse in the Bronx—and liked staying in the theater district around Times Square. So we dove into the mayhem. We checked into a hotel and caught a play that night. At a restaurant after the theater, I tried to stick with my boring diet. I didn't eat bread and I didn't order anything with cheese or pasta. I neglected to think about what was sautéed in butter or dusted with flour. Later, as I brushed my teeth, I wondered whether I should be more vigilant. I felt like I was a "sober" alcoholic who avoided vodka while giving herself a pass on beer and wine.

I shook it off, figuring trace elements couldn't hurt. Right?

Our last morning in New York, we ate forty-two dollars' worth of eggs, coffee and juice. "Ya gotta love New York hotel prices," my dad said, as we were heading out. Walking toward Macy's, we pushed through the crush of people at the confluence of Seventh Avenue and Broadway and continued a block or two before I had to stop.

"Dad, I don't feel so good. I need a cup of tea."

"OK," he said, "where would you like to go?"

I needed air, so we aimed for Bryant Park. We covered the two blocks in silence and I felt exhausted, like my limbs were heavy and I needed to sit down. At the same time, I felt my heart racing, like I'd had too much coffee and not enough food, which wasn't true. I was shaky and felt utterly alone, in the company of my father and millions of Manhattanites.

It was a beautiful April morning and people sat on the grass and at the small green tables that surrounded the big lawn behind the library. I ordered a cup of peppermint tea from the kiosk and joined my dad at a table. We sat in silence as I tried to sort out what was happening. The sun felt hot on my arms, and my feet felt like I was standing on ice. Mostly, I felt pressure, a physical force, as if all the people, sirens, car horns and conversations were pushing in on me. I could barely speak as I sat drinking the tea.

My dad sat and waited, just watching and not saying anything.

Eventually, to distract myself from this weird crushing sensation, I said, "Dad, what was it like growing up here? I mean with Grandma Ann?"

"Pretty awful in retrospect."

"Was it chaos? I mean, was there food in the fridge?"

"Oh, yeah," he said. "She took care of all that. She always kept a job. She worked in the garment industry."

"So what was so awful?"

"She said a lot of shitty things about my dad."

My grandpa Yale, my dad's dad, was one of the kindest men I'd ever met. I didn't know him long—he died when I was sixteen—but my memories are sweetness and a great Old Country accent.

When I finished the tea, we walked down to a department store on Thirty-Fourth Street. We picked a time and place to reconvene, and my dad disappeared toward the men's department. Walking felt good so I made laps in the air-conditioning, circulating through department after department without talking to anyone or stopping to look at anything in particular. Eventually, I found myself in the shoe department and bought a pair of sensible shoes, thinking that could be the answer to the persistent weirdness in my feet—just wear better shoes.

I flew back to Denver that night and slept a hard eleven hours. I awoke feeling better. The shaky energy and exhaustion were gone, same for the heaviness that crowded me from all sides. My feet, however, still felt cold. I put on my new shoes and decided I hated them.

A couple weeks later, I went back to Dr. Duncan's office. I told her about the feet, how they felt cold and tight and as if there were something wrapped around them and strung between my toes. She ordered new tests, an arthritis panel and a vascular ultrasound.

I paid out of pocket for the tests, and weeks later, when we reviewed the results, she put me on a new batch of supplements. Didn't take any away, just added to the collection growing on my kitchen counter: letters (vitamins B, D, and E) and bottles filled with glutamine, glutathione and something called IgG 2000 DF. Still, Dr. Duncan believed, the real answers lay in the heavy metal test.

"Look," she said, pulling out my results. "You have seventeen times the amount of mercury in your system."

I'd done three months of chelation and could only see the downside. "It's really hard on my body," I said. "I take the pills for three days and day four is always sucky in different ways. One day I felt weepy and couldn't stop crying. Another time I felt like I was getting the flu, that all-over achy feeling. And that day in New York, when I felt horrible, like I was standing on ice, that was day four after three days of Chelex."

Dr. Duncan told me to hang in there. She told me that several of her patients had great success with chelation. She reminded me she'd done it herself to clear up brain fog.

"How long did it take?"

"Two years," she said, "You've only just started on it. You have to give it a chance."

I said I'd think about it.

At home, I wondered about things that made me feel worse before they made me feel better. Generally, the first ten minutes of a run weren't very nice, but the next twenty or thirty were blissful. In relationships, confrontation is awful, and then it's over and the friendship or love feels stronger. Writing—the act of writing—isn't that great but having written can be heavenly.

In every example that popped into my mind, the pain-to-pleasure turnaround was pretty quick. I didn't have to wait two years to enjoy a run, a friendship or the written word. I didn't think I could stick with anything that made me feel lousy one day a week for two years.

I stopped taking the Chelex and vowed to find another solution.

CHAPTER 10

# PEACE AND LOVE ON PENDER ISLAND

On a Saturday morning, I caught the now-familiar flight to Vancouver. I'd been back twice for short weekends with Bruce since the long stay in January. I read the *New York Times* and a *New Yorker*, then watched out the window as the rich greens and blues rose and fell and rose some more until we rounded Mount Rainier. Third or fourth off the plane, I strode purposefully past the airport's "Welcome to British Columbia" indigenous plant and waterfowl display to the cavernous customs hall. The lines that fold back and forth and back again on themselves were surprisingly empty, so I continued without breaking stride up to the dark-haired customs agent behind the glass at Window No. 4.

"What are you doing here in Canada?"

"Visiting a friend."

He flipped through my passport pages. "You're here often."

"He's a good friend."

Bruce met me outside, gave me a hug and a kiss, and tossed my bag in the back of the Range Rover. He guided the car out of the international airport, around the short, squat aviation-related buildings and into the old terminal. He threw his car keys to a youngish guy who seemed happy to see him, and we walked down the dock and climbed into a four-seat floatplane. The pilot climbed in and said, "Hello, Bruce, how ya doing today?" Bruce introduced me, and we took off down the strip of water and into the air, up and over Galiano and Mayne Islands to touch down with barely a splash near Pender Island.

The pilot taxied the plane toward land and pulled up beside Bruce's dock.

"I love this," I said.

I said it every time we landed on Pender. I always felt like a Bond girl. And this always amazed me. I'm a skinny Jewish girl from Detroit, and I get to jet into Vancouver, where a handsome man meets me curbside and drives me around to a smaller plane, where we take off from the water. Twenty minutes later, we touch down and walk into that handsome man's house.

Heaven—or at least one version of it.

Ben, Bruce's seven-year-old yellow Labrador, woke from his slumber on the lawn and trotted over to meet us.

"You're looking good, big dog," I said, leaning to scratch him behind the ears. "You look like you've lost some weight."

Carrying my bag and his, Bruce caught up with us and said, "You're not the only one on a healing path. We're all getting in shape, right, Benny?"

We left the luggage on the back porch and walked around the house to the front gate. Ben trotted up ahead wagging his tail, knowing that he had a great life. He lived on the most beautiful point of the most beautiful island in the Pacific Northwest. From the front lawn, he could see Mount Rainier, and all the way around the house, he could wander among the flowers and statues of Buddha. Bruce would come and go, and Ben got to stay.

The light was beautiful and the day was warm, so without any discussion, we walked down the road past the one restaurant and onto the familiar dirt road. When we were close to the trailhead, Bruce asked, "How are you feeling these days?"

"OK," I said. "The diagnosis still scares me. I don't think he's right, but I dunno, my feet still feel a little weird."

"What does that mean, *weird*?"

"They're kinda cold a lot of the time and I feel like I can't really get a good foot plant, like they don't sink into the ground right. And sometimes, I feel like I'm wearing flip-flops when I'm not."

We turned onto the trail and started climbing, going over roots and rocks and between trees. We were moving fairly quickly, and I had no trouble navigating the terrain. "It's strange though," I said. "My gait hasn't changed, and my range of motion hasn't been limited at all. I still move the same way, which seems like I wouldn't if I had MS."

"Looks like you're moving well."

When we reached the top of the trail, we sat down on the rocks nearest the cliff a couple of hundred feet above the water. We gave Ben some water and drained the rest of our bottles ourselves. We looked out to Mayne and Saturna Islands, past them to the Strait of Georgia and over the water toward the United States.

Though sweaty from our efforts, we started feeling a chill sitting on the rocks, so we turned around, walked back to the house, opened a bottle of wine and made dinner. We built a fire and made love on the living room floor, then moved upstairs, built a fire and made love there too.

The next morning, we walked out the front gate, took the same left turn and stopped at the one restaurant for breakfast. We talked about crazy people we knew and watched a couple sitting outside.

"She's really having trouble sitting still," Bruce said, as the woman moved from one chair to another and then to a third.

From breakfast, we walked the same route to the same trailhead. We reached the top, took in the same view but didn't stop to sit; we just took a look and kept moving. On the way down, we stepped over the same roots, worked between the same trees and ducked under branches, each in our own thoughts. At the bottom, where the trail spilled onto the dirt road, we walked into full sunlight. "Bruce," I asked, "where does love fit into your life?"

I loved our weekends together and wondered why they were only weekends. And not even every weekend or most weekends. Just here and there, maybe once a month. Essentially, I was asking how I fit into his life. I'd asked some variation of the same question a few times before and never heard an answer I understood. I knew he loved me. He lit up when he saw me. When he introduced me to his friends, they'd say things like, "You're getting great reviews," or "Oh, he's crazy about you."

Bruce was silent for a bit, so I asked again, and maybe I asked again too soon.

"What?" he said.

"You know, in the scheme of things," I started slowly, carefully. "Among all the things you do and all the things that are important to you, where does love fit?"

"Why are you asking me that?" For a second, he looked young and confused. But the innocence faded and his face morphed into anger. His voice, when he continued, sounded like I had taken a baseball bat to the hood of his car. "That's not a fair question. Why would you ask me that?"

Now I was confused. There was no wrong answer. I wasn't asking to judge, just to understand. I simply didn't want to hurt or be hurt, and I wanted to understand where "we" fit in the scheme of his life, if at all. We walked along in silence until we were about quarter mile from the house and saw Jonathan and Julie walking toward us.

They were old friends of Bruce's, and he had invited them to join us for part of the weekend. They had taken the morning ferry from Victoria and had been sitting at Bruce's house for an hour or two, wondering where we were. Eventually, they decided to go for a walk to look for us.

"You look great," Jonathan said, giving me a big hug. I hadn't seen him since my meeting with Silver. I had called him though, often in the beginning. Jonathan was a helpful voice on the phone that first day. He instructed me to breathe when I couldn't and said, "One billion cells are wondering who's in charge."

I was happy to see him, though admittedly would have been happier to spend the weekend alone with Bruce.

The four of us walked back to the house, Jonathan and I talking and walking up ahead, and Bruce and Julie together behind us.

Later in the afternoon, we settled onto the big comfy couches in the living room, and Julie asked what was happening with my health.

"It's confusing," I said. "I feel the same except for my feet. I move the same. I wouldn't think anything was wrong except now, because of that stupid diagnosis, every little thing that I feel seems like some big scary thing. MS is a series of what they call 'disease episodes,' or flare-ups, with remissions in between. Sometimes when I get really scared, I wonder if I'm just in between episodes, if something is coming."

"That is scary," Jonathan said, "the not knowing."

"Yeah," I said. "Mostly I think nothing else is coming and I don't have MS. And even saying the name, MS, sounds so disproportionate to whatever's going on in my body. But the diagnosis is still on my health insurance record because all the other doctors didn't take insurance. I really want it off my record. It feels like a felony conviction that I can't appeal and never got to argue against."

"Can you see another doctor in Denver?" Julie asked.

"I don't think I can see anyone else within my HMO. I mean, I could, but I don't feel confident that anyone would have more time or would want to disagree with Silver. He's the department head, I think."

"What about Dr. Amen?" Bruce asked.

Based in Southern California, Daniel Amen works with SPECT scans, or single-photon emission computerized tomography. Instead of a flat, static image like an X-ray or MRI, a SPECT scan provides a 3-D picture that lets a doctor analyze how an internal organ works. It shows where there is activity or inactivity within the brain. Bruce had seen Amen before, to talk about attention-deficit disorder and see if Amen could suggest ways to help him focus. Bruce found the testing and the counseling that came out of it so helpful that he sent family members and some of his colleagues to California for the same testing.

"I'd love to go," I said. "I don't think I can afford it."

"That's not a good excuse. I'll take care of it," Bruce said. He could be prickly when asked to talk about love and affection, but ultimately, I realized, he had no trouble demonstrating either. His actions always felt loving to me. He liked to take care of friends and family, and I was always grateful to be in that circle.

"Thank you. That's really sweet," I said, and still felt hesitant. "I guess I don't want to go alone."

"It's a three-day exam. I can't take the time off," Bruce said and looked at Jonathan: "You want to go?"

Jonathan was happy to go and figured, what the hell, he'd get a

3-D picture of his brain too. We picked dates and set about making plans. Again, I was thankful for the people in my life. I was grateful that Bruce wanted to help financially and that Jonathan had the time and wanted to be there with me.

The next morning a floatplane came to take Bruce back to Vancouver, where he'd spend a night and then head to London for work.

I rode the ferry to Victoria with Jonathan and Julie and caught a flight from there.

Back in Denver a few days later, I checked out Dr. Amen's website, www.amenclinics.com. It explained the process of getting a SPECT scan, the reasons to do it and the risks involved. He also gave a little background on the brain:

> *The brain is the most complicated organ in the universe. There is nothing as complex as the human brain. Nothing. It is estimated that we have 100 billion neurons or nerve cells and trillions of supportive brain cells called glial cells. Each neuron is connected to other neurons by up to 40,000 individual connections between cells. You have more connections in your brain than there are stars in the universe. Also, even though your brain is only about two percent of your body's weight, it uses twenty five to thirty percent of the calories you consume. Your brain is the major energy consumer in the body.*

This insight into the brain, its volume and complexity, was exquisitely comforting to me. My brain was more interconnected and complicated than the universe—clearly no match for a fifteen-minute exam and an MRI given by a cocktail waitress in scrubs. And if there are that many connections, I wasn't sure it mattered if a few were tangled up in lesions. There are billions more ready to stand in. Redundancy can be a good thing.

And even as I was thinking of all the reasons Silver had to be wrong, I couldn't believe I was still having an argument with the guy. He was like a ghost I invited into my machine. I hadn't talked to him in months, and I knew I didn't trust him. At the same time, I was insanely shadowboxing with him and was helpless to stop.

I continued reading. Amen listed his principles and explained his philosophy:

> *When you change your brain, you change your life. By enhancing your brain function with the right treatments for your brain type, you will enhance every aspect of your life, your work or schoolwork, your relationships, your energy level, your emotional well-being, your physical health, and even your appearance.*

Amen also wrote that he didn't believe in a one-size-fits-all approach to health and that his team takes a comprehensive strategy to treat each person as a unique individual.

"We believe in skills, not just pills," the website said. "Yes, medication is sometimes a necessary piece of a complete treatment plan but whenever possible, we use natural treatments, including natural supplements, nutrition, physical exercise, targeted thinking exercises, and more. We aim to give our patients all the tools they need to boost their brain for a better life and a better body."

Music to my ears. *Medication as a last resort? Keep talking. And giving patients the tools they need? Absolutely.* The whole thing was so exciting and so promising that it was as if I had never gotten equally excited about Dr. Duncan and chelation, which I had stopped after feeling so shaky in New York.

Dr. Amen's specialty was not multiple sclerosis or anything similar. And to me, that was a good thing. I was starting to believe that we all see only what we are looking for.

So, no more MS specialists who are searching for MS only. I wanted someone who could keep an open mind and evaluate my symptoms from a different perspective.

Dr. Amen was a physician and a brain specialist, not a neurologist. Most of the conditions mentioned on the website fell under the broad category of mental health: attention-deficit/hyperactivity disorder, anxiety, depression, substance abuse and others. Amen believed that examining the brain could be helpful in treating those issues. And after doing tens of thousands of SPECT scans, he saw correlations between tendencies and regions of the brain that were either over- or underactive.

Amen also used SPECT scans to diagnose trauma and to design treatment plans using the full range of tools, like Guy Martin did at his holistic practice in Vancouver: supplements, nutrition, physical and mental exercises, and medication, when necessary.

If something was attacking my central nervous system and there were lesions to show for it, then that counted as trauma. Trauma or no trauma, if there were lesions on my central nervous system—my brain and cervical spine—then a SPECT scan should show whether they mattered. And if the scan showed they mattered and my brain wasn't working right, I liked that Amen prescribed natural treatment plans to boost brain function. He didn't say it quite as succinctly or cowboy-like as Dr. Brown—"I'm so radical, I think everything can heal"—but he seemed to be on the same page.

I read his book *Change Your Brain, Change Your Life* and thought, *All right, let's do it. If something is wrong, let's change it.*

CHAPTER 11

# I WASN'T FOUR

"Hi, it's your mom."

Even without caller ID on my voice mail, I'd know her voice, presumably the first I ever heard.

I hadn't had a real conversation with her since the diagnosis. I had mostly been avoiding her calls or taking them and talking about whatever was easy. She'd fill me in on what her husband was working on, what papers he was writing and how all his grandkids were doing. I'd tell her about the weather in Colorado.

I tried not to talk to her when I was scared. Or when I had to make big decisions. I learned this lesson when I was seventeen and not ready to go to college. I confided in my mom that I wanted to take a year off before jumping in. "You can't do that," she'd said. "We won't pay for it if you don't go now."

Dutifully, I went to college—and wound up paying my way through anyway. (I still have no idea who she meant by *we*.) In a hurry to get far away from home, I passed on the affordable state school, University of Michigan, and enrolled at Duke University. I knew the tuition was more than Michigan's, but we didn't talk about dollars in my house, and I didn't grasp the size or the significance of the difference. I followed directions, went to college, worked forty hours a week while I was there and graduated with bone-crushing debt.

Twenty years later, the debt was gone but the memory remained.

I listened to her voice mail, took a seat at my desk and made the call. How bad could it be?

"Hi, Mom," I said and started catching her up on my life. No mention of Pender, no stories of Bruce, although I did tell her about New York. I said it was great to see Dawn and meet her son and that my dad and I did well.

"You know, it's tough sometimes," I said, "to see him not taking care of himself. He's a diabetic who doesn't drink but orders a big sugary virgin daiquiri."

"You should yell at him," she said. "That's not fair of him to do to you, and you would feel better if you called your father and yelled at him."

"I don't think so..." I said and quickly changed subjects. "How's Mel?"

"He's fine. So busy. He still sees all his patients, and he's writing papers and speaking on a panel next week."

Mel's a psychoanalyst, a full-on Freudian, who married my mother when I was twenty-three and living in California. My parents had been divorced maybe six months when my mom met Mel, and they were married within a year.

When she'd told me all there was to tell about Mel, I felt I should tell her what was really on my mind. "Hey, Mom," I started hesitantly. "You know how I told you about that tingling I felt in my fingers last year? Well...I went to the doctor and now, well, actually, I've seen a bunch of doctors and there's no real agreement on what it is. One thought vitamin deficiency, another thought heavy metal toxicity, another thought MS, and another thought it was an alignment issue—you know, the result of going over the handlebars a few too many times."

I tucked the nasty one in the middle because my mom gravitates to worst-case scenarios and I was hoping to slide it by.

No luck.

"You have MS? Who diagnosed that?"

"Well, I don't know that I have it. A neurologist in Denver said it but he didn't spend much time with me, just ordered an MRI. When he got the results, he called to tell me it was MS and then really quickly wanted me to go on drugs. I don't think he's right, though, and I don't like the idea of the drugs."

"I'm here for you. You know that, don't you?"

Stunned, I thought for a second and said, "Mom, I don't know what that means."

After a moment of silence on her end, she continued on as if I hadn't said what I'd just said. "Do you want to come home?"

I hadn't lived in Detroit since I left for college and didn't think of it as home. "What would I do there?" I asked, knowing I wouldn't go. Even thinking of Detroit felt heavy, like another hundred pounds on my shoulders.

"We could get you in to see a neurologist here."

"No thanks, Mom. I've got a plan. I'm going next week to see a doctor in California and depending how that goes, I'm thinking I'll work with him or a doctor I've already seen in Vancouver who wants to take a really thorough approach to figure this out. Maybe I'll move there for three months toward the end of summer, or cousin Rona said I could stay with her in Seattle and drive to Vancouver one or two days a week."

My mom asked who the doctor was in Vancouver, and I told

her about Guy Martin. "Maybe I'll come stay with you at Rona's," she said.

"Um, you'd have to ask Rona, I guess."

"I'm sure there's room for me there."

She asked a few more questions about Dr. Martin, and I explained how I liked him and his noninvasive, drug-free approach to healing, and that I liked his commitment to helping patients heal rather than masking or managing symptoms.

"Well," she said, "it sounds like you have a plan."

"Yeah, Mom, I do," I said. "And I want to ask you something, about when you were diagnosed."

Four years earlier, she and Mel had come to Colorado for the summer meeting of the American Psychoanalytic Association. On the fourth or fifth night they were in town, over dinner, she told me she had been diagnosed with Parkinson's six months earlier. I asked why she hadn't told me.

"I wanted to wait until you could see me when I told you so you wouldn't be scared," she said.

At the time, I asked for more information, and she told me she had seen the doctor who had been her doctor forever for a routine exam, and he referred her to the leading Parkinson's expert. The expert found Parkinson's and put her on medication.

"Are you sure?" I'd asked. "Did you get another opinion?"

"Oh, no, he's the leading expert. And it's a very slow-growing type of Parkinson's, completely manageable by medication." And that was the end of the story. At dinner that night, and for the rest of their stay in Denver, neither she nor Mel had anything else to add. It was fine. She was safe. That's all I needed to know.

Now, though, years later, with my own experiences in Healthcareland, I wanted to know more.

Looking out the window, I held the phone in my right hand. "Mom," I said tentatively. "What was the symptom that led to your diagnosis?"

"Oh, I had a tingling feeling in my arm."

I felt the air leave my lungs. My head went blank. My mom and I talked for a few more minutes. And even as we were having the conversation, I could not have said what we were talking about. At some point, I recognized that she had said good-bye, so I did the same and hung up.

The conversation was too strange to contemplate. Telling me to yell at my dad, deciding to come to Rona's and then saying she'd had the same symptom but never mentioned it? And as we talked about all those things, there was an undercurrent too, something missing, words she wasn't saying and questions I didn't ask.

I put the phone down thinking the conversation went better than expected. But then, the bar was pretty low.

I called Bruce but couldn't bring myself to mention the conversation with my mom. We talked about his travels instead until I was sleepy and said good night.

The next morning, I went to a two-hour yoga class and came home, still enjoying that post-*shavasana* bliss, to a new voice mail.

"Hi, it's your mom," she said. "I talked to Mel and we don't think you should go to Vancouver. We don't want you to waste all your money on an experimental treatment with a doctor like that. He's a quack. You need to get a second opinion. If you come home, we have connections and can get you in to see the head of Neurology at the University of Michigan hospital. If you come here, we'll pay for it. Otherwise we can't help you."

Easy come, easy go, yoga-inspired bliss.

I listened to the message again.

She had seemed relatively reasonable the night before, but now, just like that, that open-minded, sympathetic version of my mom was gone and replaced with the version that gives directions without listening to the circumstances. I'd told her I'd seen half a dozen doctors to get half a dozen diagnoses. And she's telling me to get *another* second opinion?

*Oh yeah, like that one she got*, I thought.

Plus, she had no idea how much money I had or what Dr. Martin's treatments cost, and yet she knew I'd waste all my money on him. And that last bit—"if you come here, we'll pay for it. Otherwise we can't help"—I didn't remember asking for help. And, given my college experience, I suspected I'd get stuck with the bill anyhow.

I couldn't call back right away, so I just dashed off an email saying thanks but no thanks. I wished her a happy Mother's Day and said I wasn't ready to continue the conversation.

My mom did not understand.

In the suburbs of Detroit, she and Mel were celebrating Mother's Day with Mel's kids, their spouses, their kids, and my sister and her kids. They were having Sunday dinner as they'd done for so many years that they had busted out a wall and remodeled the kitchen so all sixteen could sit. I'd never been to one.

At this one, at least, my mom was thinking of me. She found time to steal away from the crowded kitchen, upstairs to the office she shared with Mel, to send me an email:

> *Thank you for the Mother's Day wishes. I will admit that I am very disappointed that we won't be talking today. After thinking about what you have told me, I would like to see you do some things before you go to Dr. Martin. It seems to me that you need a second opinion by the best neurologist available. We have resources*

*to get you to a highly respected specialist in neurology to make a proper diagnosis so that proper treatment can be started. We know the former head of neurology at U of M and you could come here to see him. Also, my Parkinson doc is a neurologist and is head of the Parkinson's and Movement Disorders Center. And we have good friends in Denver who could put you in touch with a specialist for a second opinion. I would hate to see you invest all of your savings in a questionable alternative medical treatment before exploring the best standard of medical care available.*

*I love you,*
*Mom*

"Thank you for your advice," I wrote back. "I'll consider those options."

My mom wasn't done. First, she wrote to say I was just like my father and killing myself. Lovely. I didn't respond. The next day she wrote to tell me that I would die if I didn't listen to her. I did not respond to that either. What was there to say?

On the third day without a response from me, she wrote again:

*One event you may not recall which you may want to know about was when you were about 4 years old. You were soiling your underwear and hiding the evidence in your closet. I did not know how to understand it and I took you to a child psychiatrist for evaluation. He spoke to me and your Dad and told us not to worry about it. Now I understand better that you were very angry and there was nobody to help you with that. I now believe that there must have been lots of times I didn't help you with feelings you must have had and your response was and still is to run away from those feelings just as you did when you responded to me on Sunday by telling me that you were exhausted from our conversation and didn't want to open up again. It is painful to me, also, to hear what you are going through but closing it up will not solve the problems you are having. I want to be supportive and helpful to you. I do love you.*

*Mom*

Of course I remembered it. And I wasn't four.

The intestinal distress may have started when I was four, maybe earlier, but I remember one awful experience and I was definitely five. I had started first grade without spending one day in kindergarten. Even though my birthday was three months past the deadline for enrollment that year, my parents thought I should move ahead and start first grade anyhow. Maybe they thought it was some sort of race, that I needed to start and finish school first, before all my friends, or maybe they thought I was too smart for kindergarten. Or maybe neither wanted to spend the half day with me after kindergarten ended.

For whatever reason, I was in first grade, and one night in the fall we were celebrating something; I can't remember what. My sister and I were both dressed up. I know I was dressed up because my hair was straight.

An hour or two before any event at which I had to look nice, my mom would meet me in the bathroom, wielding a hair dryer and a big, round brush. She was tall, or at least I thought so at the time, and thin. Her black hair was dark and short, blown straight to frame her small features.

My hair, left to its own devices, was complete chaos. Brown curls, with a few red strands tossed in, reached out in all directions. Some fell in my eyes; some defied gravity; and in the dense humidity of Michigan summers, all the curls gained strength and volume and went wherever they wanted.

I didn't mind. My hair and me, even back then, we had reached a happy truce. I let it do what it wanted, and it did the same for me. My mom, however, didn't love this plan. Especially when other people would see us as a family.

On those days, she'd come to the light-blue bathroom I shared with my sister. She'd clip most of my hair on top of my head and grab a section of the curliest hair from underneath along my neck. Using the round brush, she'd pull the hair straight out from my head and spin the brush under the hair and under the heat, burning my neck occasionally. When she finished the underneath sections, she'd take a fresh wet clump down from the middle and work that. When the middle sections were dry, she'd start on the top layers. One section at a time, she'd pull the hair, spin the brush, and point the hot air, over and over, until forty-five minutes later, when my once-crazy curly hair lay down flat and pin straight, shiny all the way to ends.

Sometimes it hurt. Always it was hot. And while I didn't enjoy the process, I endured it. I was getting attention from my mom, and she did some version of this to her own hair every day.

For this celebration, with my hair straight and shiny, I sat with my sister in the backseat, belted in, while my dad drove and my mom rode shotgun. My parents went to fancy restaurants, nightclubs or concerts every Saturday night while Ellen and I stayed home watching TV with the babysitter. This must have been a big night, because we were included.

The restaurant had white linen napkins and older male waiters who acted as if they'd never seen kids before. The menu was full of foods I'd never tried and words I didn't know.

"Could you tell me how the lamb is prepared?" my mom asked the waiter.

"What do you recommend, the sweetbreads or the duck?" my dad asked.

My father ordered for all four of us, and soon a team of servers set the first wave of plates upon our table. If the Campbell's soup and grilled cheese sandwiches we normally ate were food, then these dishes, drenched in heavy sauces and exuding rich, warm smells, were some otherworldly delicacy, created for luxury, not sustenance.

My parents were sharing a bit of their world with us, so my sister and I dug in and tasted everything—appetizers and breads, entrées and desserts—as if we could prove we belonged by enjoying this food, as if our enjoyment was something we could give our parents. We ate until we could eat no more.

When all four of us were completely stuffed and all the plates and silver was gone from the table, the waiters returned with tinfoil swans of leftovers that they presented to Ellen and me. We giggled and said good-bye, walked outside into the heavy air and took our seats in the family sedan.

"Why do we buckle up?" my dad asked, mimicking some public service announcement. "We buckle up for safety."

Ellen and I did as told and my father guided the car onto city streets. We'd gone less than a mile when I felt a grinding in my belly. My family talked about the meal and the restaurant and the waiters, and I sat quiet and withdrawn, hoping the pain would stop. When it didn't and I could take no more, I said, "Dad, I think we have to stop. I have to go to the bathroom."

Ellen sighed an exaggerated sigh like a big sister would, and my mom turned to look at me. "Couldn't you just make it home?"

"I don't think so."

My dad pulled into the parking lot of a Howard Johnson's, and my mom and I ran inside. We sprinted past the hostess stand to the bathroom. I barely got inside the stall, locked the metal door and pulled my pants down before an explosion came out of me. Like the food at the fancy restaurant, this awful mess came in waves.

After the first, my mother asked, "You ready to go, honey?"

"I don't think so."

After the second wave, I heard her say, "Could you flush the toilet, Jody? It really smells." And after the third, she said she'd wait outside.

Keeled over in pain and confusion, I leaned forward on the toilet, my stomach resting on my cold, skinny legs, while I stared at the tile floor. I wondered when this might end and how it would end.

Eventually, it just did. The eruptions subsided and I pulled myself together. I met my mom in the hall and we walked back to the car, and all four of us drove home in silence. No one asked how I was feeling or what had happened. It was almost as if it hadn't happened or we had reached a silent agreement: if we don't talk about it, it didn't happen.

While I didn't understand the silent strategy, I was the kid of the family, and figured they all knew more than me. And I was used to it. As a family, or even one-on-one, we didn't talk about things that were painful or embarrassing or ugly or confusing. And diarrhea hit on all four of those.

But the incident after the fancy restaurant wasn't the first. Or the last.

In first grade there were more than a few episodes of intestinal distress. My stomach hurt so often that I was a regular in the nurse's office. On occasion, I went to see the nurse because sitting in class, I'd feel that grinding in my belly, and before I could figure out how to get out of the room and down the hall to the bathroom, I'd have what my mom called "an accident." Afterward, I'd go to the nurse's office overcome with shame and fear.

One time, I went to see the nurse and started sobbing uncontrollably. My face filled with tears and snot and humiliation. The nurse, a kind woman with a round face and round glasses, handed me a box of Kleenex. I just looked at it, uncertain what to do.

When I cried like this at home, my dad would say, "Please stop crying. I'll give you a dollar if you stop." I'd be crying and crying and crying and he'd beg, "Please stop. Just stop, please."

The nurse, however, seemed fine with my outpouring of feelings and wanted to help with the snot. She pushed the box closer to me and I took a tissue. I held it between my fingers around my nose and squeezed tight as if I were about to duck underwater. Then I blew until my cheeks turned red.

"Oh, honey," she said. Her face softened into an easy smile. "Sweetie, you have to leave a little room. Don't hold so tight. Leave space so you can blow the snot *into* the Kleenex."

She showed me how. I tried again and it was a revelation. I was amazed that my parents had never shown me how helpful Kleenex could be. *Maybe they didn't know*, I thought. *Wow, this is something I can show them.*

But by the time I got home I had forgotten my new trick, or maybe I just knew if I brought it up I'd have to tell why I was in the nurse's office. As we passed canned peas and roast chicken at dinner that night, my dad asked each of us, as he always did, "How was your day at school?" I said what I always said: "Fine."

I avoided any discussion of these episodes until it wasn't possible any longer. Some weeks later after a particularly messy accident, the nurse told me to wait as a neighbor, Mrs. S, who lived across the street from us, was coming to pick me up, since my mom was working. She gave me a bath, threw my clothes in the washing machine and loaned me her daughter's clothes to wear. Then she sat at the kitchen table and drank milk with me while we looked at the trees in her backyard. She asked questions, and I told her that art was my favorite class at school.

I wondered what it would be like if she were my mom.

When my real mom knocked on Mrs. S's front door, I said goodbye and walked home with my mom in silence.

She didn't mention the episode that day or the next—or the one after that.

Eventually, however, I experienced the same intestinal distress with a similarly messy result.

That night my mom yelled at me for it. "You had another accident. Wasn't it enough that Mrs. S had to come get you, and now she knows about this? Why do you do this? It has got to stop."

She gained volume with every word. I looked around for an escape, but no one came for me and, at that moment, deep inside my five-year-old brain, in the part that controls the fight, flight and freeze instincts, I suddenly came to understand that I couldn't flee; I couldn't fight. I could only freeze, and I was alone. I was the only hope I had, and no one, not even my mother—especially not my mother—was going to wrap her arms around me and tell me that everything was going to be all right.

And everything was not all right. Whatever was causing contortions in my belly, it was not all right. It hurt, and it was something to be ashamed of and something to be hidden. I couldn't tell the neighbor because, although Mrs. S. was incredibly kind, my mom thought it was horrible that she knew. And now I couldn't tell my parents because my grief and pain and bodily functions caused *them* so much pain and anger that it looked like they might break apart. And that was no good. I couldn't have parents who were in pieces. I was only five.

Weeks later, after I got home from school, my dad came home early, changed out of his suit and the three of us (my parents and me) got in the car. I was wearing my favorite shirt, blue with horizontal red stripes, warm and snugly like a hug. In the car, I thought something special was happening—my dad came home early, and my parents were taking me somewhere. *We must be going somewhere good*, I thought, so I asked where.

"We're going to the doctor's," my mom said.

I thought of Dr. Miller, the pediatrician we saw when my sister or I threw up or spiked a fever. "But I'm not sick," I said.

Neither replied.

When we got to the doctor's office, I saw that this guy wasn't Dr. Miller at all. He had no stethoscope, tongue depressor or silly jokes. This guy's office had shelves of books, a big desk and a couch. There was no glass jar with cotton balls and no white coat. My parents waited outside and the "doctor" asked me to sit on the couch.

He wore a blue button-down like my dad wore to work and a tweed jacket with elbow patches. I wondered about those. He had a soft face that wasn't unkind, light brown hair and wire-rimmed glasses. He introduced himself to me and asked how I was.

"Fine."

He didn't ask what I'd been eating or how my belly felt or anything like that. He leaned across his desk to get a better look at me, small in my striped blue shirt, sitting on his big leather couch. "Jody," he said, slowly. "Do you have accidents?"

"Nope," I said. My mom told me that I should be ashamed that Mrs. S knew. Why would I tell this guy?

He saw right through my lie and asked why I had accidents. I stared at him without moving, thinking it must be a trick question. I mean, if I knew why I had them, I could avoid them. They were "accidents," after all. Didn't he know what an accident was? That it was something you didn't do on purpose?

"Nope," I said again. When my lips came together on the letter *p*, I resolved that they would stay that way. I did not trust this man. I would not speak to him. I crossed my arms over my chest, tucked my chin and stared at a spot on his chin.

He asked another question. I listened and stared. He asked one more, and I listened and stared some more. Eventually, he recognized the futility and said, "OK, now I'd like to speak to your parents."

The doctor opened the door to let them in and I sat down in the waiting room, which had a short table and matching kiddie chairs, covered in coloring books and crayons. From the big window, daylight flooded the room.

When the door opened again, my parents came in and the doctor said good-bye. With my parents, I walked back down the hall, into the elevator and outside to the car. The three of us got in, drove home in silence and no one ever mentioned the trip again, leaving me to wonder what it was all about or whether it had even happened at all. Sometimes I thought I just made it up. But I knew the drill. It had happened, but in my family, if we don't talk about it, it didn't happen.

I went back to school the next day and the day after that and sooner or later, I learned to sit still even as my stomach churned and raged. I learned to clench all the muscles in my back and belly so nothing made its way out of my body until I was in the bathroom with the door safely locked. Over time, I got so good at gripping the muscles around my guts that I didn't even notice I was doing it.

I became so skilled at ignoring distress signals sent from my stomach that I thought it was normal, something everyone did all the time. Certainly it was nothing to mention or complain about.

## CHAPTER 12

# AMEN TO THAT

Jonathan and I landed at John Wayne Airport and rented a car to drive the half mile to the Amen Clinic. (It's California. People drive everywhere.) We had appointments that afternoon, so with our luggage still in the car, we took seats in the waiting room. Before long, a social worker came to get me.

She had long, dark hair, and clear skin and large, dark eyes. She looked young. And kind—she looked kind. She showed me to her office, told me a bit about herself and asked if I had questions. I didn't, not right then.

"OK," she said and added three unrelated words. We talked a little more about the clinic and how long she'd been there and, after a few minutes, she asked if I remembered the three words. I did.

Then she opened a file with the fifteen-page questionnaire I had filled out and faxed in weeks before. There were questions about mood swings, sleeping patterns and eating habits. There were questions about my childhood, who I leaned on for support, how often I felt stress and how I handled it. I told her I didn't have a problem handling stress. And I believed it.

The social worker went through the pages, confirming some

answers and asking about others. When we got to the stress section, we spent a lot of time talking about the MS diagnosis. I hated how it was delivered. I hated how I reacted to it—by canceling a trip I had been looking forward to. I hated the doctor who gave it to me, and I hated him more when he wouldn't answer my questions or return my calls.

And still, I was scared he was right. I wanted it ruled out. I asked if the doctor who would interpret and review my SPECT scans could do the same with my MRI. She said sure, so I gave her the CD.

The interview continued as she asked about my friends, my family, my lover. I told her about Bruce and how he did amazing things like supporting me through this adventure in health, that he was paying for the brain scan I was about to get. And that even though he took care of big things like that, it made me a bit sad that he wasn't available for simple things, like a Sunday brunch or a midday call. She seemed to understand why that would be hard, and she seemed so empathetic, so friendly, that I wanted to ask her about her own relationship, like we were friends chatting over coffee.

We weren't. She was a social worker gathering information about me and my brain. She asked me to count backward by subtracting seven at a time from one hundred. After a few minutes she stopped and asked for a number.

"Thirty-seven," I said.

She then asked about speeding tickets and traffic accidents, how often I experienced déjà vu and whether I remembered those three words again. I did.

I thanked her and went back to the waiting room, curious about what she'd learned from asking me to remember three words and count backward. A few minutes later, an imaging technician came to get me. He explained how the SPECT scan worked and told me what to expect. The first day, he would inject me with a radioactive isotope, called a tracer. When he took the pictures with the SPECT scan, the tracer would highlight areas of blood flow.

We would take two sets of images: one after I'd played a game on the computer and another after I'd sat quietly in a calm, dimly lit room. We would do the same two images on the second day without the tracer.

"In very rare cases, the isotope causes people's urine to turn green," the tech said.

*That's awkward*, I thought.

He set me up in a small office to play the game, and after ten minutes, he came to take me into the imaging lab. It was a big, open space, well lit with none of the creepy, claustrophobic feeling I'd gotten from the MRI cave five months earlier. The tech was in the room with me, not behind dark glass sitting at a desk and conferring quietly with another person who was never introduced. And the machine itself was less intimidating than the MRI.

I didn't have to change my clothes or remove anything to get started. I just sat on the table and lay back to rest my head in a small cradle. I focused on my breathing and lay still while the imaging device moved around my head like the moon orbiting the earth. The camera made a gentle hiss as it glided from one position to another and the tech stood by, checking in with me from time to time.

I zoned out a bit, fell into a nearly meditative state, and then was surprised when the tech told me we were done. "See you tomorrow," he said as he walked me back toward the waiting room.

"How'd it go?" Jonathan asked when he reappeared a few minutes later.

"Pretty easy," I said. "How about for you?"

"Same," he said.

That night over Korean food, I asked about urine. "He said it could turn your pee green," I said. "Mine was leprechaun green, not just a little, but bright, bright green—like the greens at Pebble Beach. Was yours?"

"No," Jonathan laughed. "He said it's really, really rare for that to happen."

"I must be special."

We talked about the schedule for the next day and what we each hoped to learn from this adventure. I said I wanted to rule out MS and learn what was happening in my brain.

"And before we go, I really, really want to walk on the beach," I said. "We're so close, and I need to walk on sand."

"No problem," Jonathan said. "We can go when you're done tomorrow."

On the second day the scans were just as easy, maybe easier. In the evening, Jonathan and I drove south on the Pacific Coast Highway until we found a beach that looked like a good long walk.

I immediately took off my shoes and stepped into sand. My feet felt like they'd been sprung from a cage; my toes freed from solitary confinement. "Ooh!" I squealed. "This feels so good. I'm so happy here. My toes feel like we've descended onto a whole new planet."

"Oh, so this wasn't just about seeing the water and the sky?" Jonathan said.

"No, this was a therapeutic outing," I said. "I don't know why, but for months, I knew my feet needed the beach. The weekend that we all spent on Pender, I'd been trying to get Bruce to meet me somewhere warm, with a beach, but he couldn't make it work."

After an hour or more of walking, my feet felt completely rejuvenated—and with them, my heart. The flip-flop feeling was gone, and each toe and each little bone in each foot felt like it was moving independently and easily. Before we walked back to the car, Jonathan and I sat on the rocks to watch the sun go down. It was stunning and inspiring, relaxing and reassuring, as California sunsets always are.

We found a restaurant where we could sit outside to see and hear the ocean. We shared a table with some French tourists, and we each trotted out our limited language skills.

"*Bon appétit,*" we said when the food came.

"Enjoy your dinner," the Frenchies said.

The next morning, I went back to the clinic to meet a doctor who had reviewed my questionnaire, MRI, social worker's notes and SPECT scans. I asked Jonathan if he would come too, just in case.

Dr. Arsalan Darmal is a diplomate of the American Board of Neurology and Psychiatry and is board-certified in child and adolescent psychiatry. He had dark hair, wore a suit and looked to be in his fifties. He sat with us around a coffee table and handed me two pictures of healthy brains.

One looked like a Claymation model, sculpted in pastel-colored Play-Doh. The other looked like an engineer's line drawing, with blue lines showing the outside structure and red and blue lines creating shapes inside.

The Claymation brain, which Darmal called the 3-D surface image, showed activity on the surface. A healthy brain is symmetrical with a smoothish surface. Unhealthy brains, Darmal said, are uneven or pockmarked or asymmetrical.

The engineer's drawing Darmal called a 3-D active brain image. It showed activity in the brain. Black spots mean no activity. Blue means a medium level of activity. Red means high activity, and white means super high. The cerebellum, which is involved in motor control, balance, coordination and cognitive functions, should be red and white, showing very active neurons. The rest of the brain should be mostly blue.

Once I'd had a moment for the images of model brains to sink in, Darmal gave me pictures of my own brain. Handed them to me, gave them to me, mine to keep. And unlike the hazy gray images of the MRI, these things looked like a brain. My brain. How weird.

The Claymation one, with its light greens, pinks and yellows, was mostly smooth and looked symmetrical to me. No holes or missing parts. I was pleased.

Darmal, however, saw something not quite right in the right and left temporal lobes, which can be associated with moodiness, irritability, memory problems, abnormal perceptions, anxiety, spaciness, headaches or abdominal pain.

As he rolled through the list, I mentally crossed or checked off each item. My mood did ride up and down often—which I attributed to blood-sugar surges and dives—and abdominal pain was a fairly common occurrence. I didn't think I had memory problems, but maybe I just didn't remember them. Mostly though, I'd been ignoring all these symptoms. I thought they were normal and it hadn't occurred to me that they didn't have to be.

"This could be related to trauma," he said.

I thought of Martin saying I was more trauma than illness. And again, I wondered, *What trauma?* I'd never broken a bone, never been hospitalized, never been to a war or experienced physical assault.

"You also have mild decreased activity in the prefrontal cortex, which has to do with attention and motivation," he said.

This triggered something deep. I'd always thought I was an underachiever, that I couldn't focus or stay motivated.

I looked at Jonathan. "Breathe," he said.

I really didn't want another doctor to tell me there was something wrong with my brain. Until this moment, despite flying all the way to California to have someone examine my brain, I hadn't admitted to myself that this could be a possibility.

Partly, I'd been blocking out the potential for more bad brain-related news. And mostly, leading up to this appointment, I'd been focused pretty tightly on the email exchange with my mother, putting my house on the market and evacuating it for repeated showings. I was busy with work too, finishing another assignment for a nonprofit.

When I thought about coming to California, I'd thought of it almost as vacation, with the added bonus of getting another medical opinion from another angle. I'd assumed that this new opinion would correspond completely with my own thoughts. I don't think I said this out loud, or even silently to myself, but I figured at the Amen Clinic, someone with fancy diplomas would tell me that yes, I was right, and Silver was wrong. I assumed the doctor would say there was no way I had MS.

As Darmal talked about the imperfections he saw in the Claymation model, I began to wonder whether this whole trip was a bad idea. I didn't say anything. That horse had left the barn. I couldn't get up and walk out—what would be the point? Darmal moved on to the other picture of the brain—the red, white and blue drawing—and pointed to two white spots on the top of my brain.

"These two often come together," he said. "They are like cousins, anxiety and depression."

Darmal waited a moment for that to register. "You've probably been dealing with these for a long time," he said. "Maybe you didn't even know you were dealing with them."

"Well," I started, thinking of the recent anxiety- and sadness-inducing conversation with my mother. There had been others, too many to count. "That may be," I said. "I remember when I realized that not everyone needed to spend time lying on their bed staring at the ceiling. I thought that was normal."

He almost smiled. I looked at Jonathan. He looked calm.

"And," Darmal said, "your cerebellum is a little lazy. I'd like to see more activity there."

*Great, and now I have a lazy cerebellum too?*

Darmal didn't seem so disheartened. In fact, he felt like the pictures showed a pretty healthy brain and that with proper exercise and nutrition, my brain could function even better. The good doctor moved straight to solution.

"With your brain chemistry, you need aerobic exercise where you get your heart rate up for thirty to forty minutes at least four times a week," he said.

"I can do that," I said. And truthfully, I'd been feeling a little sluggish lately, like I needed more exercise.

"Also I recommend supplements, fish oil a thousand to two thousand milligrams a day, coenzyme Q10 and a vitamin B complex once a day," Darmal said. "And vitamin D3, five thousand IUs a day until you get your level up and then go back to two thousand IUs a day."

He also suggested that I take phosphotidylserine, a component of cell membranes, and a GABA receptor, which would help reduce anxiety.

Finally, he suggested yoga and meditation, and if balance was a concern and I wanted to work on it, he said I should try *Dance Dance Revolution*.

*Fish oils and vitamins B and D? Check, already on 'em. And meditation? Got that going. It wouldn't hurt me to spend more time in a yoga studio, and* Dance Dance Revolution*? A Nintendo game? Fabulous.*

"I can do all these things," I said with a cheerleader's enthusiasm that my next thought quickly quashed. "That's great…What about the MS?"

"I'd rule it out," Darmal said. "I looked for a long time at the MRI, trying to find demyelination, and I saw only a little evidence of it. I think the anxiety and depression are the real issues for you. If you're worried about the demyelination, you can try a hyperbaric chamber. They've had good results with that."

"I don't have MS?"

"I don't see it. There are areas of your brain that need to be cooled off and others that need to increase their activity for you to feel your best," Darmal said. "The program I've outlined for you here will help. Do you have any questions?"

"No," I said. "I don't think so. I might later. Well, I guess I do. So just to be clear on the MS…"

"Yes, I can see how that's stressful for you, and given that anxiety is an issue for you…But no, I wouldn't worry about it. The diagnosis was premature. I don't see it. Don't worry about it. Just take care of your brain."

And with that, I couldn't think of anything else to ask. I packed up my notebook, filed the photos of my brain back in the ring binder he gave me and stood up to leave. Mentally, I was already celebrating the fact that another doctor with a wall full of fancy diplomas checked my MRI and four more descriptive pictures of my brain; thoroughly reviewed my medical history; ruled out MS; and prescribed fish oil, yoga and a video game.

"Start with the supplements I've prescribed, and if those don't help with the anxiety and depression, you might want to try Lexapro, an antidepressant," Darmal said. "Make a phone appointment and let's talk in six weeks."

I shook his hand, thanked him profusely and floated out into the Southern California sun.

Jonathan and I hugged in the airport and boarded flights to go our separate ways.

The next day in Denver, my suitcase lay unzipped near my closet with clothes and shoes spilling onto the floor. I didn't want to unpack because I didn't want the trip to be over.

I loved California every time I had gone, and on this trip, I had checked off the top items on my wish list: a respected medical specialist said it was not MS and prescribed yoga, meditation and nutritional supplements; the sand massaged my feet; and Jonathan and I enjoyed great conversations.

I started to sort the laundry in my luggage but then stopped. I wandered into the kitchen to put on water for tea and went into my office. I fired up the computer, opened my email and found a note from my mom. I had almost but not quite forgotten about the nastygrams she'd sent before I left town. I'd almost but not quite buried the memory of my mom bringing up an incredibly humiliating incident from my childhood, telling me that I was killing myself like my father, and that I would waste all my money if I went to the doctor I liked.

I was already sitting at my desk looking at a message without any words in the message bar, just "No subject" next to her name. I considered deleting it unopened and didn't.

*We have been at this place before and I am done with it. I am furious at the way you treat me. While you are not responsible for my feelings, you are responsible for your behavior, which is about the meanest way I have ever been treated by anyone. You are cruel and selfish. I will not put up with it. I am through feeling sick and depressed.*

I sat still and listened for my breathing. I couldn't hear it over the loud whistling that sounded like a train coming through my house. It took a moment to remember the teakettle.

I walked into the kitchen and turned off the stove and set the kettle aside. I found my phone and called my dad. I told him about her note and waited.

"All those years, I was public enemy number one," he said. "Now, it looks like it's you, kid."

"I don't even know what she's talking about," I said, "What did I do that was so mean? Get diagnosed? See different doctors? Not see her doctor?"

I forwarded the email to him while we were still on the phone. I hoped I had misread it, that I was missing something that he could explain.

He took a minute to read her words and said, "Has she gone off her medications or something?"

"What?"

"Something must be wrong with her," he said.

"Yeah, she's cruel. That's what's wrong."

"C'mon, Jo. Don't say that. She's your mother."

We got off the phone, and I took my dog outside for a walk to clear my head. As Riley and I wandered the neighborhood, I wondered how my mom could interpret my health scare as something I was doing to hurt *her.* Also, how long she had been "feeling sick and depressed," and how often had she blamed me?

Riley trotted along wagging her tail, as if her default mode was joy and she needed no reason to be happy.

Maybe my mom's default mode was anger. For all those years and all those events where she was angry at me—my childhood stomachaches, my college graduation, my marriage and divorce, and now this—I always wondered what I had done wrong. Maybe the answer was nothing. Maybe she was angry first and found fault with me second to give reason to her rage.

When I got back to the house, I answered her email as thoughtfully as I could, explaining that I didn't understand what I'd done to hurt her and that I hoped she could understand that I was scared too and also needed kindness.

I didn't hear back.

CHAPTER 13

# BIKES AND HAMMERS AND NAILS

I owned a beautiful bike. Black, sleek and strong, it was built with carbon fiber and California cycling genius. It was a gift from Bruce and weighed nearly nothing. For several months, it had been standing against a wall, looking neglected.

Three days after I flew home from the Amen Clinic and two days after I said so long to my mom, I pumped up the tires, found a pair of cycling shorts and filled a pair of water bottles. My loft downtown sat two blocks from the nexus of an eighty-mile system of bike paths. I had no excuse. I hopped on my bike and rode along the South Platte River. I pointed toward Chatfield Reservoir, which would be thirty-eight miles round trip, though I knew there was no way I would reach that today.

I rode for twenty minutes before I needed water. Uncoordinated, and not confident enough to pedal and drink, I stopped the bike and pulled over. I took a long pull on my water bottle and realized I was done for the day, or I would be soon. I turned around to head for home. First day: forty minutes. Not epic but not bad.

One fine day, I'd make it to Chatfield. In the meantime, I wrote "Bike 40" on my calendar and colored it green.

The next day, I went to the yoga studio and wrote that in my calendar in green too. I planned to ride every other day and practice yoga in between with one day off each week. If I wrote it down and color-coded it in my calendar, I'd have no way of convincing myself I'd been exercising if I hadn't. There would be ample evidence in green or there wouldn't.

At the Amen Clinic, Darmal had prescribed exercise and meditation. The good doctor said my brain needed both, so I promised myself six days of one and seven of the other each week. I'd been sitting nearly every day since December. In the beginning, ten minutes seemed an eternity and, simultaneously, a throwaway event. You can do anything for ten minutes, I'd tell myself, as if the time were inconsequential. Then Darmal told me there were consequences, and good ones at that: better brain health! This was the treatment plan. Exercise and meditation were medicinal, and they were medicine I could live with. No side effects, no scary pharmaceutical companies and no contrived research studies. Meditation had history on its side—thousands of years in dozens of cultures. I bumped the timer on my meditation app up to twenty minutes.

After four weeks of daily meditation and bike-yoga-bike-yoga-bike-yoga, I added another five minutes to the meditation and distance to the rides.

One afternoon, I pedaled along the Clear Creek Trail from Denver to Golden, a fifteen-mile stretch with a four-hundred-foot climb at the end. As I pushed up the incline, I thought about Martin, whom I still had an appointment with the following week. Originally I'd thought I'd move to Seattle or Vancouver for three months of treatment with him to see what he could do. Now it seemed unnecessary. And a bit dramatic.

The conversation with my mom may have had something to do

with my change of heart too. But I hoped I had reconsidered only because relocating seemed like something I'd do if I were really sick. And I wasn't. Dr. Darmal said so.

As I struggled up the path around North Table Mountain, I pulled my water bottle from its cage, drank a bit and poured some over my neck and back. For the twelfth day in a row, the temperature hovered in the nineties and I chose to ride at the peak—late afternoon when the asphalt sends as much heat up as the sun sends down.

I pedaled and reviewed the previous six months and the doctors I'd seen. I wondered whether I'd been running in circles and knew the answer was yes. I'd been running from doctor to doctor saying some variation of "Can you fix me?" It seemed pathetic, and yet I understood what drove me. The tingling felt strange and stuck around, so I knew it meant something, the way a persistent runny nose could mean allergies or a worsening cold. I wanted to know what caused it, and Silver's explanation had terrified me, as much for its finality—MS is permanent—as for its unpredictability—waves of symptoms come and go, each one worse than the one before until the game is over.

And Silver was the lone voice on the record that health insurance companies used to determine rates. The other doctors told me it wasn't MS, but since I paid out of pocket, they didn't automatically make notes in my record, and none gave me an official-looking letter declaring me disease-free. In the world of insurance companies it was my word against Silver's, and he had medical degrees.

In the real world, however, the one that existed all around me as I pedaled onward, I decided I was going to be fine. I looked down at the computer on my handlebars. Ninety-some degrees on an incline and I was still tooling along at sixteen miles per hour. Not bad.

*I'm better than fine,* I thought. *If I were broken, and really needed fixing, I couldn't handle this hill or this heat.*

Then, of course, I heard it. "On your left," some guy yelled. Two guys in matching jerseys powered past me as if I had two flat tires and was hauling a trailer.

They made it look easy, almost effortless. And that is the blessing and curse of living in Colorado. The place is lousy with endurance athletes. Everywhere you look, there's some guy who rode in the Tour de France or won the Leadville Trail 100 mountain bike race, or there's some woman running six-minute miles while pushing a baby stroller.

A few years before, I had taken my dog for a hike to Silver Dollar Lake. I drove through Georgetown, over Guanella Pass at eleven thousand feet and along a winding, one-lane dirt road. Wearing hiking boots and a baseball cap, I brought water for me and Riley, snacks for both of us, a topo map and sunblock. On the trail, I stepped over roots and logs and rocks while Riley bounded over and through it all. About ninety minutes into this hike, I'd built a solid sweat, even Riley was starting to slow down, and we saw two women coming toward us on the trail. They were moving quickly with minimal gear. No backpacks, no water bottles.

When they came closer, I could see that they were muscular and tan and beautiful in that rugged, outdoorsy sort of way. They were probably in their sixties, and one was wearing sports scandals and the other Birkenstocks. Aging hippy chicks were killing me on the trail.

On my way to Golden, I smiled at the memory and pedaled a little faster.

When I was putting my bike away a few hours later, the phone rang.

"How ya doing, Jo?"

"Pretty good, Dad. How about you?"

We talked for a while, and he caught me up on my sister and her kids. He asked if I'd talked to my mother, and I said I hadn't heard from her since the last exchange.

"How's your health?" he asked, moving the conversation along.

"It's fine. I feel fine. I've been riding my bike a lot—went for a good ride today. I have a little bit of tightness in my feet but whatever. I don't know if the lesions are still there or if they even matter," I said.

"Yeah, it's hard to know," my dad said.

"This whole thing just seems crazy. Like Silver saw me coming, and since MS was the number-one diagnosis he gave women like me, he sized me up, checked off a few boxes—woman, young, athletic—and declared MS. Then he couldn't take my calls questioning his wisdom."

"I remember when I took your grandfather to the Mayo Clinic," my dad said.

This sounded vaguely familiar. My grandfather was a big, strong man with powerful hands. He was a plumber and built his strength carrying porcelain tubs on his back up flights of stairs.

"What was wrong with him?"

"It started as a tingling in his feet, and he lost power in his legs," my dad said, as if we hadn't been talking about my tingly fingertips for nearly a year.

"It got so bad he couldn't work," my dad went on. "It took us forever to get an appointment with the neurologist, and when we finally got one, I flew in from law school to take him there."

I'd never heard this story before. My grandfather was probably in his late fifties at the time, and I wasn't around yet.

"The doctor finally arrives with a harem of residents," my dad said. "He walks in and says, 'Mr. Berger, I'm going to refer you to an orthopedic surgeon. You have a pinched nerve in your neck.' I said, 'Wait a minute, you haven't even examined him.'"

My dad continued: "The doctor says, 'OK, Mr. Berger stand up. Close your eyes.' And my dad's spinning like a top. The doctor says, 'OK, you can sit down. Were you standing straight?' My dad says he was. The doctor says, 'Look over there,' and he pokes him in the leg with a pen and my dad doesn't even feel it.

"One of the residents says, 'And you should see his walk.' The doctor looks at the resident like he's the biggest bag of shit he's ever seen, but he says, 'OK, Mr. Berger, could you walk for me?' And his walk is horrible. He was losing power in his legs."

My dad tells the story as if this were just another story. As if I hadn't been terrified this whole time by tingling. He tells the story of my grandfather calmly, without emotion other than amusement.

"The doctor says, 'I'm going to refer you to an orthopedic surgeon. You have a pinched nerve in your neck.' We took him to the Mayo Clinic. He had the surgery and his health improved until he was in his seventies and the symptoms came back. At that point, they wouldn't do the surgery again." My grandfather worked until he was nearly eighty and lived until he was nearly ninety.

We hung up, and I sat there dazed. I tried to read. I tried to watch TV. I woke Riley, told her she needed a walk, attached her leash and headed outside.

When we got home, I thought about all the doctors and all the stories.

The doctor with an MRI machine and a self-proclaimed proclivity to diagnosing MS found MS. The traumatologist found trauma. The neuropsychiatrist found anxiety and depression. And the doctor with faith in a heavy metals test found heavy metal toxicity.

Add in my family history of tingling in the extremities, the leading expert in Parkinson's found Parkinson's in my mother and the doctor who claimed he didn't even need to examine my grandfather to know what was wrong with him found exactly what he said he would find: a pinched nerve.

Maybe instead of bouncing through all these doctors, I should have started with a psychologist like Abraham Maslow. He's the guy who explained the law of the instrument this way: "To a man with a hammer, everything looks like a nail."

CHAPTER 14

# TOES AND TEETH

In late September, I rode into the Chatfield Reservoir and, feeling the strongest I'd felt in a long time, considered taking a right to Bear Creek State Park. Turning around and heading back the way I came meant nineteen more miles. Taking the right would add ten more for a total of forty-eight on the day. I pictured the provisions in my pockets and on the bike: a couple of energy bars, a packet of Shot Bloks, keys, cell phone, two water bottles—one half full with water, the other half full with an electrolyte drink. I had plenty of fuel and there were plenty of places to grab water if I needed to.

I took the turn and started heading into the sun. The fall air felt cool on my arms and the sun warm on my face. The great grassy areas were mostly yellow, and the late afternoon light bathed everything in warmth.

On a bike, I covered so much more ground than I did at a run, mentally and physically. The rhythmic spinning of the pedals was almost meditative, allowing my feet to do the work and my mind to wander freely while another part of me, a calmer part of me, could simply sit back and observe its path.

As I cruised toward Bear Creek, my mind wandered down to my

feet, which still felt different than they should. They felt constricted, like something was wrapped around them with something stretched between my toes, but neither was the case. The phantom constraint and flip-flop sensations were only slightly uncomfortable, but I still wondered why I felt them.

I'd had similar curiosity over a different new sensation—the fingertip tingling—which had launched nearly a year of doctor searching. As I pedaled, I thought, *I can live with my feet like this*, and maybe the cause of the sensation was less important than what happened next. I was on the bike, happily pedaling forty miles further than I pedaled only months before, and so my next thought was about Dr. Darmal at the Amen Clinic. Right after I got home from California, I pedaled for twenty minutes and had to hop off to take a drink and then turn for home because I was tired. I tried again a few days later and every other day after that though, because Dr. Darmal had told me to. He looked at pictures of my brain, listened to my complaints and told me to exercise thirty minutes at a stretch for four times a week. He didn't spend a lot of time trying to explain the reasons for the features he saw on my brain pictures or how those features created symptoms or led to my complaints. Instead of telling me a chain of events that could have led to my appointment, he used the appointment to tell me that in his experience, and Dr. Amen's experience, certain features often appear with certain symptoms. He talked correlation and didn't spend too much time on causation. And he said, in his experience, that he also saw correlation between certain actions—exercise, meditation and vitamins—and a lessening of symptoms.

Correlation or causation? Always an interesting question, and something I'd pondered a lot on this medical odyssey. Initially, I went to the doctor to find the cause of the tingling. Silver said he found it on the MRI: the lesions caused the tingling. But what caused the lesions remained a mystery. I didn't get to ask Silver, but I often wondered how he knew which way the arrow pointed. How did he know the tingling hadn't caused the lesions?

And now, as I pedaled into the sun, my body served as physical proof that my own actions could improve performance. As if I hadn't learned that in my years as a sportswriter. I'd seen hundreds of athletes go to their coaches and work together to design a program that incorporated exercise, nutrition and motivation, to make the athlete better, faster, stronger, more balanced, more fluid or more of whatever they needed. I'd also seen plenty of athletes work with their coaches to overcome injury and illness. In the athletic world, poor health, good health and high performance sit on a continuum and the magic mix of exercise, nutrition and attitude is a constant lever to move a person along the continuum.

As I thought about all the athletes I'd interviewed and all the coaches they'd praised, I realized that that was the relationship I'd wanted when I first went to the doctor's office. I just hadn't thought about it before I made the appointment. If I had, I might have asked for an expert to run some tests, listen to me talk and take a general inventory so he or she could say, "Here's where you are now, at point A, and here's where you want to be, point B, and with my expertise and experience I will design a program to get you there."

Instead, I told my story to the first expert, Dr. Wise, who listened, saw my symptom as someone else's responsibility and referred me to a neurologist. Dr. Silver ran some tests, listened to my story and took a general inventory, only to say, "You're at point A and all I can do is offer you different drugs to prevent you from sliding backward, to some scary negative point D."

We weren't playing offense—designing a plan of attack to move me forward—we were playing defense, considering drugs to keep me where I was. And on the defensive play, I would not be an active participant. Other than paying for and injecting the drugs, I wouldn't have much of a role in this really important part of my life. If something I was doing had contributed to the tingling, I'd continue doing it unaware, as if my actions had no impact on my health—good or bad.

This didn't make sense to me. Why forgo offense and settle for defensive medicine, where the goal is only to slow my decline? The only reason I could think of was a certainty that offense was impossible, that there was no potential to move toward better health. And that didn't make sense to me either. Of course, good health can be fleeting. But can't poor health be temporary too? Why do so many of us believe that good health is fleeting and poor health permanent?

✚ ✚ ✚

After I got home from the ride, I went to the Tattered Cover, a great, locally owned bookstore with comfy chairs, strong coffee, two floors, and shelves and shelves and shelves of books. I didn't know exactly what I was looking for, only that I was thinking about coaching, training, exercise and how the body adapts. Isn't training the thing that allows the body to do something in September that it couldn't do in June? If training can cause the muscular and cardiovascular systems to grow, adapt, change and develop, why not the nervous system too? Why would something so critical to growth and development and change not have the same healing capability as the rest of the body?

I wandered among the tables and aisles of books on the first floor. I read book jackets and checked out the author photos. I scanned the shelves and read the store recommendations taped below them. When I got to the table of new nonfiction, there it was: *Mindsight*, by Daniel Siegel. I'd never heard of the book or of him, but I liked the cover.

I dropped into the nearest chair and read the introduction. "Mindsight has the potential to free us from patterns of mind that are getting in the way of living our lives to the fullest," he wrote. Siegel explained "mindsight" as a way of focusing attention on the mind to see clearly the way we think, feel and behave. "Interestingly enough, we now know from the findings of neuroscience that the mental and emotional changes we can create through the skill of mindsight are transformational at the very physical level of the brain," he wrote.

I bought the book, brought it home and reread that section. I reread and reread the lines he wrote explaining how the act of focusing attention can serve as a "scalpel we can use to resculpt our neural pathways, stimulating the growth of areas of the brain."

As a physician looking to improve his patients' lives, Siegel focused on mental activities that would enhance their health. Intrigued, I also wondered whether the opposite was true, if thoughts, feelings and focus could tamp down pathways or slow growth in the brain. Anyone who's been so sad that their stomach hurt understands that emotions can cause a physical sensation. Could emotion also leave a physical mark? Could emotional trauma cause lesions? I don't know that the research has ever been done. I wondered whether Siegel would touch on that and kept reading.

I read about Siegel's patients, including a teenager and an elderly gentleman who learned to practice mindfulness, and by doing so, changed their brains and changed their lives. And finally I read about a woman who decided at the age of eleven that she would not feel again. Her father was absent and her stepmother unkind. One day, after feeling hurt for what seemed like the hundredth time, the woman, as a young girl, decided that it had to stop. She couldn't change her parents so she changed herself. She committed to not feeling the pain again.

Years later, she went to Siegel because she couldn't feel anything at all. She hadn't just numbed out the pain. She had numbed out everything. She was smart and successful and numb. Siegel wrote about how she couldn't handle her feelings of loneliness as a kid so she chose to freeze them out. She couldn't fight or flee, so she went with freeze.

Over time, freezing out her feelings—good and bad and everything in between—became habitual. I pictured her and wondered what decisions I made as a kid that had become habitual, what choices were so routine that I didn't even notice that I was still making them. Specifically, I wondered whether my experiences growing up were now affecting the decisions I made about my health and my interactions with doctors.

I sat down on the couch and reviewed my medical history. I pictured myself as a five-year-old wracked with stomach pain. The "treatment" for this problem eventually seemed to be shame, embarrassment and a bewildering trip to a shrink, rather than something to address my physical ailment.

I thought about earlier and later doctor visits too. Before I could walk, for example, my mom thought my feet turned in too far and rushed me to a doctor, who said, "Ooh, you got here just in time. We can fix her," and explained how to screw my baby shoes to a metal bar.

Years later, after the stomach-churning incident, one doctor thought my exhaustion might be the sign of something permanent and fatal but then later said, "Oops, didn't mean to scare you. It's only mono."

And then there was the really terrifying event, which started when I was eleven. I was in seventh grade and my mom took me to see a pair of orthodontists. They were a father and son team whose office was about ten minutes from our house. Both men had brown hair—the son had more of it than the father. Neither man was tall, although the son came closer. The father wore glasses and had cheeks that chipmunked out when he smiled. The son was better looking in a nerdy sort of way.

"You have such little teeth, and such a small mouth," the old man said as he poked around with a mirrored tool. "Please, open your mouth wide," he said. "And close. Now open. And close."

I sat in the big chair of peach-colored leather, or maybe pleather, and tried to ignore its cold, creepy feel. I heard the humming and whirring of dental drills and suctioning things, and smelled that awful mix of antiseptics, mouthwash and ground teeth while the two men examined me.

When they'd seen all they needed to see, the son filled my mouth with gunk that felt, smelled and tasted like Silly Putty. It sat heavily like a blob on my tongue. When the putty set, the doctors had their mold, and I could rinse and spit in the sink. Then the dad orthodontist brought my mom in from the waiting room.

"There's not enough room in your mouth for all your teeth and your tongue, so we'll extract four teeth and create some more space," he said to me, I think, although he was looking at her. "We can move the teeth with braces to create a better smile and healthier bite. We'd like to get started right away."

I wasn't sure my teeth were tiny or that my mouth was too small or that any of this was a problem. They were my teeth in my mouth, and I had no trouble eating or smiling or talking so the whole set up worked for me. No one asked me though, and the experts thought something was wrong, so why let the situation get any worse?

In short order, I lost four teeth, lived on soup and applesauce for a few days, and healed just in time to go back to the orthodontists. On the second visit, my mom took a seat in the waiting room and settled in to read while the assistant showed me back to the big peach-colored chair, where I sat tipped back, looking for at least an hour at the non-glare lamp hanging from the ceiling. The dad orthodontist sat on one side and the son orthodontist on the other. They had me open my mouth as wide as I could, so wide that my jaw hurt and my neck ached, so wide that I wanted to scream but couldn't because four hands were jammed inside my mouth—which at this moment, as they had said, felt tiny. They poked between my teeth and nicked my gums and jammed metal rings onto my molars.

When they had shiny cold steel circling all my teeth, the orthodontists went to work with an industrial-smelling glue, wires and pliers. There was more cranking and twisting and poking. I wished I could be somewhere else. I wished I were someone else. My sister didn't have to do this.

I didn't cry but could feel my eyes were glassy and unblinking as I sat, trying to breathe, staring at the reflection of my own teeth and tongue in the dad orthodontist's glasses.

When they were finished, the two men escorted me back to the waiting room, had me smile to show my mom a mouth full of metal and told her I might experience some discomfort. "You can give her some aspirin to help her sleep," the dad orthodontist told my mom, as if I no longer spoke the language.

That night, in bed, I remember thinking, *They don't know what discomfort means.*

The first night with orthodontia is "discomfort" in the way an eighteen-car pileup is a fender bender. For me, the searing, cutting pain seemed most intense when I lay down and couldn't find any place for my head. I couldn't rest on my back, or on either side, and sleeping on my stomach was out of the question, because that meant my neck would twist and one side of my jaw would have to be in contact with something.

Little by little, night by night, the pain would lessen and I'd get more moments of sleep until about a month after the injury. I could finally sleep through the night, just in time to go back for another round. My mom would pick me up from school and take me back to the office building where father and son would probe my mouth and crank on the wires connecting all my teeth.

After a few of these monthly sessions, the orthodontists fit me for a neck gear—a scary contraption that attached to my back teeth and pulled the upper half of my smile toward the back of my head. It hurt like nothing I'd ever known. It felt like it was crushing my brain and forcing all twenty-nine bones in my head to rearrange themselves—which of course it was.

After a few months with the neck gear, the orthodontists decided I needed another device. The upper half of my smile was not only too far forward; it was too narrow as well, they said. My tongue was squished. I hadn't noticed the problem, but they seemed certain that my tongue needed more space, or it would someday. A palate expander was called for. While I didn't know what this was, I knew it couldn't be good.

Powerless, I sat in terror, with my eyes wide and tearing, as the two men fitted me with a metal bridge that crossed the roof of my mouth and attached to two teeth on either side. There was a hole in the center of the bridge and a teeny key that fit into it. Every night I was to turn the key, which would push the bridge apart, widening the metal across the roof of my mouth, splitting my upper jaw and rearranging, yet again, all twenty-nine bones—pushing them apart from the inside.

If I had thought I'd never know any pain greater than the neck gear, this beast was a rude awakening. This thing hurt like the world was ending. And the worst part was I was complicit. The pain was self-administered. The orthodontists and my mother said if I didn't turn the key, I'd have to wear this thing longer, so I turned the key. Like them, I feared that something worse would happen if I didn't crank it a notch every night. It didn't occur to me that nothing could be worse.

Every night I felt my head exploding. Sleep was out of the question and food looked like pain. I wore the palate expander, cranking it wider and wider, for months. And I went to school every day like I always did, although instead of sitting in the front and raising my hand to ask questions, I sat in back and tried to see over the pain in the center of my head, the center of my universe.

And then thankfully, thankfully, one fine day, the orthodontists told me it was done. The palate expander accomplished what they wanted it to achieve, so they removed it. I went back to being a kid with normal ugly braces on all my teeth.

Months later, the orthodontists told me the whole thing was done. They were ready to remove the dreaded bands. The two orthodontists organized their instrument trays and started the procedure, using a pair of pliers to yank the bands free from the cement they had used to secure them so long ago.

My mom sat in the waiting room reading, and I held my mouth open as wide as I could for as long as it took. And the removal seemed to take as long as the installation, but I didn't care because this was the end. This was it. No more pain or suffering for a better smile.

The dad orthodontist took me outside to show my mom my new smile.

"Ooh, that's great, Jody," she gushed. "They're beautiful. How do they feel?"

"They feel great. Let's go."

She made an appointment for a follow-up in one month. I said good-bye and we were gone.

One month later we returned, and the orthodontists had me sit in the peach chair and put me through the old drill, "Open, close, open and close." I was watching them from such close range that I could see nose hair. And I could see that their expressions did not show joy. They looked concerned. Or worse.

The dad orthodontist went to the waiting room to get my mom. When they returned, he said, "There's still not enough room. She has such a small mouth, and well, her tongue is going to move her teeth over time."

I stared in terror and panic and confusion. I held my breath.

"What are you suggesting?" my mom asked.

"Well, we'd like to put the bands back on, and since we've gone as far as we can with the palate expander, there are other options to discuss."

The son orthodontist stood silent.

"One thing we could try," the dad orthodontist said, "is to shave down the sides and tip of her tongue."

Now my eyes widened even more, and I screamed. "No way," I said. "No. Way."

And finally everyone looked at me as if they just remembered I could speak.

The dad orthodontist tried to talk me into tongue surgery. It's not that big a deal, a minor, minor surgery—really, just minor. The son orthodontist nodded as if his dad were very wise. And someone said something about how this might sound bad now but it could prevent worse problems in the future.

The way I saw it was this: I had suffered through two years

of pain they had designed specifically for me, and now they were saying that all my suffering didn't matter, that it didn't achieve their intended results. And, they added, if I knew what was good for me, I would submit to more.

I'd fallen for this once—this story that "there's something wrong with you and we can fix it but only with extreme measures. So do as you're told and don't question the experts." Two years later, I wasn't so gullible. "No way," I said. "No way. Uh-uh." I unhooked the bib the orthodontists had snapped around my neck, put it on their instrument tray, climbed down off the chair that no one had lowered back to the ground and walked out of the office. My mom met me near the drinking fountain in the hall and we left.

In the car, my mom drove and I stared straight ahead at the faux-wood finish on the dashboard. I had a vague notion that the sky was clear and that the radio was not on. I couldn't articulate what just happened. I didn't have the language to explain that two experts had tortured me for two years and, without admitting their incompetence or asking my forgiveness, then had determined the experiment a failure and asked for another shot at me.

And the next time, they weren't just going to come at me with pliers and drills and wires. They wanted to come at me with knives. They wanted to cut off my tongue.

I think the lesson I took from the experience at the time was: do not trust medical professionals to know what's best and always double-check their suggestions. The lesson probably stayed with me subconsciously through my appointment with Silver and into Vancouver, where I panicked when Christopher and Guy wanted to have a meeting about me, without me. But luckily, new information leads to new understandings.

At thirteen, I thought the orthodontists were out to hurt me.

Three decades later, I think they were probably doing the best they could with the tools they had. They just didn't have very good ones. They didn't think to ask the kid what she wanted or what she was willing to do to get there. Neither my mother nor I knew to ask their plan or goals, and we didn't know how to evaluate either option. We all assumed that their idea of best outcomes and acceptable trade-offs matched mine—or that their ideas were the only ones.

As a kid, I was angry that no one consulted me. Three decades and a half dozen doctors later, I understood that a doctor couldn't possibly point me toward my goal if I wasn't clear on the goal myself. And if the doctor didn't consult with me, it was up to me to make sure I was heard anyway.

If I were to see another doctor, I'd want her to work with me like a coach might. I'd want someone to understand that I'm at point A, want to get to point B and need to take an active role—working with my body, not against it—to achieve results.

I was sure doctors like that existed—I'd met them in Canada and California. There must be at least one in Colorado too.

## CHAPTER 15

# MEXICO WITH MITRA

As September rolled into October, I was still riding my bike, practicing yoga and seeing Bruce when I could. My feet still felt strange, and I wondered whether it was neurological in nature or related to the lesions, but I chose to continue researching it on my own for the time being, rather than see another doctor. (I'd already seen so many!) Inspired by *Mindsight*, I collected books on brains and healing, with titles like *The Brain That Changes Itself*, by Norman Doidge; *Perfect Health*, by Deepak Chopra; and *How Doctors Think*, by Jerome Groopman.

I also wanted to reclaim that trip to India, so I emailed Mitra and asked if she were taking students again and when. She wrote back to say she had no plans for India but was taking a group to Troncones, Mexico, in November and I could join them.

Of course I went.

The first morning in Mexico, just before eight o'clock, I unrolled my purple mat onto the hardwood floor. Above me was a thatched roof held aloft by rough-hewn posts that looked like young and naked trees. The walls were nonexistent. From where I stood, I could see the pool and six bungalows around me and the beach and ocean before me.

I inhaled the warm coastal air and looked over the sand to watch the Pacific curling in on itself and racing toward me and then away, toward me and away. I shut my eyes to listen and realized that even without seeing the water, especially without seeing it, I could feel its relentless and replenishing power. I stood with my eyes closed, breathing and listening, until I heard people join me on the hardwood under the thatched roof.

"Take a comfortable seat," Mitra said, bringing me back into the *palapa*. Everyone had arrived. All six students were present. Class was about to start.

We sat down cross-legged facing our teacher and, behind her, the ocean. "We will practice yoga twice a day," Mitra said. "And I will ask you to journal and share your thoughts with each other."

The six of us sat upright, with our backs straight and our eyes perked like puppies, looking happily to our leader for love and direction.

"I will ask you all to be intentional," she said. "We are here for a week, and today I will ask you to write about your intentions, what you hope to do here."

Then Mitra introduced the first chakra, which is located at the base of the spine and governs survival, security and passion. And she led us through a series of poses designed to energize that chakra. Mostly, we lay with our backs on the floor, working our lower bodies, lifting one leg up and out to the side, then the other, then both legs straight up and holding them there until we heard Mitra's voice: "And down you come."

As we worked our lower extremities, Mitra said more about the first chakra and told us what Mother, Mitra's spiritual teacher and a student of Sri Aurobindo, said about survival, security and passion. As we strained minute after minute after long minute to hold each pose, working against inflexibility and incoming fatigue, we listened to Mitra say, "Little by little," except from her mouth, the words were softer, sweeter and the *T*s weren't really there. It sounded more like, "Lillel by lillel, your hips will open."

At the end of the two-hour class, she had us lay flat on our backs with our legs long on the floor for the final time in *shavasana*, the corpse pose. In this resting pose, the body and mind integrate all they have learned in the hours leading up to the pose. My limbs felt heavy and happy as I inhaled the warm, coastal air and listened to the water racing toward me and away, toward me and away. I felt tears rolling down the sides of my face, and I realized they had been gathering and growing under my eyelids until they found their way to the corners of my eyelashes and rolled to freedom. They were happy tears. I realized I too felt free, and I was overcome with gratitude.

After class, I met Mitra in the little beachside restaurant for breakfast, and before everyone else arrived, I told her I had cried in *shavasana* because I was so grateful to be right where I was. And as I told her, I started crying again because I knew it was true. As strange and scary as my crazy journey of diagnoses and misdiagnoses through the health-care system had been, I was grateful for all that I was learning. I knew I was on the right path.

"Thank you," Mitra said. "Thank you."

After breakfast, I walked on the beach, wrote in my journal and walked the beach again.

At about three in the afternoon, I was walking back to my little bungalow and saw Mitra sitting in the pool. From anywhere near the pool, you could see the ocean. On one end of it, the wall came up toward the surface of the water then flattened out for a couple feet so we could sit on the ledge in six inches of water. I sat down beside

Mitra and finally told her in detail why I had to cancel the India trip nearly a year ago, in January.

I hadn't seen her in person since then and didn't check in with her again until I was ready to put the whole episode behind me and try for India one more time.

At the time, I said yes to Mexico and didn't go through the whole story of my medical odyssey. Even if I had wanted to, email seemed inadequate. And for whatever reason, I hadn't thought to call.

So, sitting in the pool in six inches of water, looking out toward the Pacific, I took what felt like the first chance to tell her what had happened to me.

And I told the story in its entirety. I told her about the tingling and how it came and went and how I didn't think it was a big deal. I told her how Silver said I should get the MRI before I left the country and how the MRI tech hassled me about what the contrast dye cost and how she said using dye was so unusual. And I told Mitra how scared I was and how badly I just wanted to get to India so I could relax.

Sitting nearly hip to hip in a swimming pool under the warm sun, I told Mitra how, after the MRI, I was home organizing my gear to pack for India when Silver called to say I had MS. I told her how scared I was, how I couldn't breathe.

Without a second's hesitation, Mitra wrapped her arms all the way around me, really hugged me with force and love and strength, and said, "Oh, baby."

Her movement was so swift and so sure and so powerful that I realized this was all I wanted. A big and certain hug with a heartfelt "oh, baby"—this is what a mother does instinctually, and this is what I had wanted my mother to do. This is the way a mom tells a child that she will survive, that she is safe.

This is what I wanted when I was five years old and my stomach ached. This is what I wanted when I was thirteen and the orthodontists threatened to shave down my tongue. And this is what I wanted when I graduated college with a mountain of debt and no clue what to do in the world or how to pay it all back.

And mostly, this full-body hug with a simple, straightforward, sincere "Oh, baby"—this is what I wanted my mom to do when Silver told me I had MS.

Until this moment with Mitra, I had no recollection of an experience like this, an embrace so strong and supportive that I knew I would survive. And without any knowledge of a hug like this, I didn't know it was what I wanted and I didn't think to ask. When I told my mom what was going on, I didn't feel held in response. I felt pushed away, and still I kept emailing her, kept trying to convince her, because I was still her child and still believed, unconsciously and despite all evidence to the contrary, that my mom could deliver.

As I sat sobbing and unwinding in Mitra's arms, Mitra delivered—she held me and held me—and it felt like the first time anyone had ever done this for me. Mitra's hug and love felt so nurturing and, at the same time, so foreign to me that I sat bewildered and unwilling to let go of this full-body, completely emotional and totally unconditional love.

With the sound of the ocean over my shoulder, and this small Iranian woman wrapped around me, I felt so good and so safe and so reassured.

"Oh, baby," she said, and that was all. "Oh, baby."

After a while, we had more to say, but we didn't stop hugging or crying.

Mitra and I sat holding each other and sobbing and talking as I told her the rest of the story about my adventures with the callous people at my HMO and the lovely, caring men in Canada. I explained how I was so desperate to figure out what was really wrong with me and cure myself that I got a 3-D picture of my brain in California, discovered Deepak Chopra's book, and decided I'd like to learn more about Ayurveda because it sounded like a more holistic and gentle way to assess what was going on with my body.

"Oh yes!" she said and again, her accent was so fun that *yes* almost rhymed with *race*, although the one-syllable word had two beats and sounded like "yay-es!" when Mitra said it.

Still hugging and sitting hip to hip in six inches of water in a lovely little swimming pool under the full sun in Troncones, Mexico, we laughed and talked and cried until we were finished. We didn't rush or even realize whether anyone had come near us. We just stayed in the conversation until it was complete, and when it was, we learned that the hour had slipped past four o'clock, closer to four thirty. We jumped and scrambled back to our rooms to change clothes because Mitra had a yoga class to teach and I had one to take at four. *Whoops*...

We reconvened in the gorgeous, wall-less yoga studio near the water.

Ninety minutes later, my limbs once again felt strong and my lungs felt large. When we lay down in *shavasana* for the second time of the day, I was again overcome with gratitude because I knew I was exactly where I was supposed to be. There wasn't a chance in the world, no matter what anyone said or whatever was happening anywhere else, that I was meant to be anywhere but in Troncones with Mitra and the five women who were laying on their mats all around me. There was nothing I was supposed to hear other than the powerful Pacific, and there was nothing I was supposed to feel other than the warm wind coming off the ocean.

That night in my bungalow, I fell asleep listening to the soft whir of a ceiling fan and the subtle clicking of geckos talking to one another.

In the morning, I went back to the *palapa*, eager and energized. For day two, Mitra moved to the second chakra, which is located just below the belly button and governs creativity, emotions and sensuality.

"Water is the element associated with this chakra," Mitra said. "It concerns flow and movement."

And with that, Mitra led us through two hours of forward bends and cobras, downward dogs and puppies. At the end, in *shavasana*, my mind was nearly clear. I could hear the ocean and nothing else. No thoughts, no self-talk, nothing, just ocean.

After class, all of us migrated to the café and ordered eggs, fruit and coffee. We talked about the class we had just completed and classes we had taken before. Two women in the group, Beth and Diane, had gone to India in January when I didn't go. As they talked about the time they spent there, I felt regret that I hadn't been a part of it and comfortable enough to tell them why I wasn't.

"I wish I had gone," I started, "but at the time I was so scared. As I was organizing my stuff to go on that trip, a neurologist called to tell me I had MS."

Six women at the table all looked suddenly and intently at me. None looked scared. None looked like she pitied me or felt sorry for me. Each one of them, still wearing their yoga clothes and their post-*shavasana* calm, looked at me with interest and openness. They looked like they cared and wanted to know what happened.

So I told them. I told them about Dr. Silver and the doctors in Canada and what I learned about vitamins B and D and their impact on the nervous system. I told them about how I felt in my body and how my mind churned in terror.

I talked to these women like I had known them forever, and I felt I had. I told them how scared and helpless I felt dealing with each doctor in Denver and how empowered and excited I felt working with doctors who believed that healing was always possible.

"How did your father handle it?" Beth asked.

"Really well," I said, somewhat surprised by the question. "He was great, wanted to clear his schedule and come with me to Vancouver." At the table, all six faces brightened to hear this. "It was my mom who didn't do so well," I said and watched their expressions lose the light.

Three of the six women at the table were mothers and all of us, we all had mothers.

"At first, on the phone, my mom seemed to be tentatively listening, but then the next day she seemed to change to say I was doing everything wrong and that I had to fly to Detroit to see her doctor. When I said no, it sent her spiraling out of control. One day she was like, 'You've brought this on yourself because you don't share your emotions with me.' And the next day, 'You're just like your father and you're going to die.' And finally she said, 'How could you do this to me?'"

Six women gasped in unison. "What?" Diane asked.

"I know, it was so crazy that it kinda snapped me out of my stupor. I had been trying to have a conversation with her, trying to negotiate to get what I wanted, and when she said that, it was like, 'Well, I can't do this right now. I have to focus on my health.'"

Around the table, over the half-eaten plates of fruit and scrambled eggs and avocado, I saw six faces in various phases of anger and sadness. And on all of their faces, I saw kindness and care and concern. And I saw a desire to help, a wish to be with me on this journey and to make sure I knew I was not alone. And I wasn't. All of a sudden,

I knew I wasn't. I had big sisters and little sisters and maybe moms too. Even though they weren't my mom, they were moms, and they knew how to do the mothering thing. They just sat with me, listening to me, not jumping in to offer advice or criticize or condemn. They were just present, sitting at this table in this moment, listening to me and being with me as I recounted a really terrifying time in my life.

And we sat at the table until the conversation was complete. No one rushed. No one looked at her watch or made an excuse to get up from the table. I felt supported and loved and accepted. And for the fourth time in two days, I was overcome with gratitude.

By day five of this Mexican yoga retreat, we were all so close to one another that we were sharing passages from our journals as if sharing our most private thoughts and fears was no big deal, as if we did it all the time, without fear and without judgment. We were becoming the people we wanted to be, bigger, stronger and braver. This transformation seemed to be happening inside of five days, but I knew the process of growing healthier in mind and body had started months earlier.

Later that afternoon, back in my bungalow, before our second class of the day, I grabbed my cell phone and went to the restaurant to take advantage of the wireless connection. I'd been checking my email once a day, deleting or ignoring all the notes except ones from Bruce. He was also in Mexico, at his new house in Cabo, and we were checking in daily.

I typed a quick reply to him, told him how grateful I was to be right where I was, surrounded by the ocean and warm air and fabulous feminine energy. I wrote that I loved him and hit "Send."

Then I scrolled through the rest of the emails and found one from my mom.

*Hello Jody,*

*I keep thinking about you and how much I miss you and then I realized that although you are my daughter, I don't really know you. Nor do I think you know me. Can we "meet" and get to know each other as we are now?*

*I love you,*
*Mom*

I hadn't had heard from her since May. It was now November. (Granted, I hadn't contacted her either.) Six months had passed in such radio silence that I'd figured it might be permanent.

Ignoring all the emails that had come before it, her email said she loved me and wanted to see me. My gut response was gratitude. Instinctually, I started crying and ignored the guts of her message: she said she didn't know me, after forty-three years.

I was so grateful to get word from my mother and so into this heart-opening Mexican adventure that I brought my phone to our next class and read the email out loud. A big, sweet "aw," came back at me from all sides. Everyone was happy and relieved that my mom had reached out to me. I was too. I was hopeful.

The next morning, I brought my phone into the wireless zone and sent my mom a note saying I was in Mexico with limited access to email. "Call me next week," I wrote. "I love you too."

That day, in class, Mitra taught about the sixth chakra, located between the eyebrows and often called the third-eye center. The sixth chakra is associated with compassion, clarity and the inner vision that gives us the ability to discern the truth and see the past, present and future.

After class that morning and the next day, I reconsidered the message from my mom. Surrounded by love and compassion and nurturing motherly energy, I realized I wasn't ready to go home and wasn't quite ready to face my mom.

We had a long history in which we'd built a clear pattern. Often when we talked, I felt unheard, misunderstood or dismissed, and she may have felt the same. I know she often felt hurt, like I was purposefully trying to upset her (though I never was). The email exchange about MS was only the most recent (and most upsetting) example of the two of us failing to connect. As I reread her last email, I wanted to believe that we could change in an instant and feared we couldn't. I didn't want to relive the past and wondered how our future relationship could be different. I wanted to lock myself into the perfect present where I was sitting: surrounded by love and warm ocean breezes with an invitation to kindness from my mom.

As beautiful as the picture was, it was still temporary; eventually we all had to leave Troncones. Two cabs carted all of us through the dark, lush landscape that eventually gave way to two-lane roads and then four lanes to the airport. And once we had all checked in and cleared the security line, we hugged good-bye and kissed and hugged again. We talked about having a mini-retreat or reunion in California soon. I waved as they boarded the flight to California and I waited alone another twenty minutes before beginning my trip back to Denver.

In Colorado, the air was cold and the sun was strong and my schedule was full. I had lots to do in the two weeks before I was to fly back to Mexico to spend Christmas with Bruce. My mom called, and when I saw those three letters on my iPhone, MOM, I cringed. The last time we communicated had hurt so badly that I was still hesitant to reopen that conversation. I feared I wouldn't get to say what I wanted and needed to say, that we would hang up feeling unheard, misunderstood or dismissed.

I wasn't ready to connect live over the phone, so I sent an email. It seemed safer, like an electronic olive branch testing the murky waters between us:

*Hi Mom,*

*I've been thinking about you and the email you sent. I do love you and miss you and, at the same time, it's painful for me when we interact.*

*A while ago, you wrote that you were overwhelmed with your anger towards me. And that's true for me too.*

*A number of big life events—when I got married, when Hugh and I threw a party, when I got divorced, and most recently and most painfully, when I was having health challenges—seemed to go through the same pattern. Each time, I thought I'd feel compassion from you, and instead, I felt your anger. I don't know why. I do know the amount of anger I feel from you is overwhelming to me.*

*This last conversation, in May, around my health issues, was the turning point. I really don't understand your response and your anger at me then and I can't pretend that didn't happen. If you want to explain it to me, that'd be good. If not, I understand and I'm going to keep my distance for a while.*

*Love,*
*Jody*

I hit "Send" and waited.

No response arrived.

It was disappointing. As difficult as our relationship was, my mother wasn't a bad person; we just disagreed on how to move forward. She wanted to start over as if the past never happened and I couldn't do that. The past *had* happened. Through a series of small decisions, made over time, we had built an unhealthy relationship. I'm sure both of us wanted it to be better, to be loving and thoughtful, and yet we couldn't get there in an instant.

The same was true for my own health. I made a series of small choices over time that resulted in me going over the handlebars, running on adrenaline and eating in a way that, meal by meal, left me low on vitamins B and D and eventually probably resulted in this insistent tingling. Getting to a better place, physically and in my relationship with my mom, would thus have to be a similar campaign—nothing instant but a steady plan, taken choice by choice, day after day. And that's where I determined to start.

CHAPTER 16

# GO FIND ONE

Bruce and I woke to the sound of the ocean and took a long walk on the beach. His family was coming in a few days for Christmas, and on this gorgeous day, we were alone, just the two of us.

We walked side by side, sinking into the sand with the waves crashing to our left, free-associating and talking about this and that, about nothing and everything. With New Year's looming ahead, I looked back on this year of doctors and didn't need any special expertise or self-awareness to see how I'd spent my time.

"I've been obsessed with my health and as much as I'm sick of going doctor to doctor and listening to all kinds of theories on what's wrong with me, I also don't want to fear doctors for the rest of my life," I said. "Or think the only good ones live in Canada or California, because that can't be the case."

Bruce smiled, and we started walking again. When we reached the big rocks at the end of the beach, we turned around and started walking back to where we had started from forty-five minutes earlier. We walked along in silence, each in our own thoughts until I said, "My New Year's resolution is to find a doctor I trust, not because I may have MS or may not, but because I want a doctor who knows me and is nearby. I want someone who looks at the whole picture."

"So find one..."

The first week of January, I did. Deepak Chopra's book, *Perfect Health*—in which he explains Ayurvedic medicine, one of the world's oldest healing traditions, which looks at the body, mind and spirit as one integrated whole—had resonated with me. I searched for an Ayurvedic doctor and found Nita Desai, a Boulder physician who runs East West Integrated Health. I called to set up an appointment and started to fill out the extensive paperwork she requested. I answered questions on my diet, my sleep habits, my stress load and how often I "eliminated" excess food—which took me aback, since I'd learned as a kid that no one should ask or talk about that kind of stuff. She asked me to keep a food diary for three days to see what my diet was like and to list any medications, allergies, or past emotional or physical traumas. She also asked for any and all test results, saying that she often saw the test results in a different light and analyzed them differently than other doctors.

On a blue-sky day, I left my home in Denver and started up the road to Boulder. Ten minutes into the twenty-five minute drive, the sky turned bluish gray, and I was glad I'd thrown a jacket in the car. Ten more minutes and the sky grew darker still, and I wished I'd thrown in a hat and gloves too.

Snow was starting to fall when I found her office. I checked in with the receptionist and looked around. The waiting room was barely big enough for four chairs, the water cooler and a small bookshelf. An illuminated rock sat on the floor next to the water cooler and a framed photo of open bags of brightly colored spices hung on one wall.

I looked at the books on the shelf and smiled. She had *Perfect Health* too.

After a moment, Dr. Desai came around the corner to take me back to her office. A small woman, no taller than a sixth grader, she had short dark hair and looked to be my age. A taller, younger, dark-haired woman was with her and asked if she could join us.

"Hi, I'm Victoria, a fourth-year medical student. Would you mind if I observe?"

"Of course not."

Inside her office, Dr. Desai flipped through my records in the standard manila folder with two holes punched at the top that every doctor seems to have. The difference was that the folder was already fat, and this was our first meeting. I knew they were the pages I sent her, and still, as she flipped through them, I got a little nervous and my palms began to sweat.

Dr. Desai asked questions calmly with a completely neutral face, showing neither approval nor disapproval. She asked about the initial symptoms. She was the first doctor who was actively interested in the abdominal distress that had started long before the tingling. She asked about the tingling, so I told her it had started in my right hand, jumped to my left and, after the steroids, landed in both feet too.

I told her that I'd pulled or torn something in my hip, which made the heel-toe walk part of Silver's evaluation really challenging. "I think he thought this was a neurological symptom, and I think it was related to the hip joint being out of whack," I said.

I told the now-familiar story of how he spent fifteen minutes with me, ordered an MRI, called me at home and told me I had MS. And at this, Dr. Desai looked up from the pages in her lap. She looked to me and then to the med student, who seemed equally surprised.

"Victoria is closer to medical education," she said. "Aren't there asymptomatic lesions—lesions that show no symptoms of disease?"

"Sure," Victoria said. "Often. In fact, many perfectly healthy people have asymptomatic lesions that aren't indications of any medical problem. They're just there."

And for the first time, I was thrilled to have a medical student in the examining room too.

Dr. Desai continued, "There are studies about lesions..." but I was so excited I couldn't wait for her to finish her sentence.

"I know," I said, even though I didn't know. I had just thought and hoped this was the case and the lesions didn't matter and that lots of healthy people had lesions. "I wanted to ask Silver if you took one hundred people off the street, how many would have lesions. But I could never get a hold of him to ask that or any other questions."

And then I almost relaxed and we rolled on through the interview, asking and answering questions on diet, exercise and the effects of the Prednisone.

"My symptoms got worse," I said. "I'd only had tingling in my extremities, and all of a sudden it was a full-body experience, starting at a spot in my low back and radiating out. I have a meditation practice but couldn't find calm while on Prednisone."

Dr. Desai nodded again. "That's the Prednisone reaction. It's common."

Then she looked at my food diary and asked about breakfast. "Is that instant oatmeal?"

"Yes."

"And lunch, what's in the salad?"

"Spinach, tomatoes, maybe some goat cheese."

"Uh-huh, and how many times a week do you eat chicken or fish?"

"Two, maybe three."

She frowned. This didn't seem to be the right answer.

"How often do you have a bowel movement?"

"I don't know," I said, "every couple days."

Judging from the look on her face, this was definitely not the right answer. "You need to eliminate every day," she said.

"People do that?" I asked, disgusted.

Dr. Desai nodded and continued with questions—nearly an hour and twenty minutes worth—until she said, "Now, I'll do the exam. Can I see your tongue?"

I showed her my tongue. She made a note and looked at my face, drawing lines on a small outline of a face on her page. She then held my right wrist to check a number of pulses, looking down in deep concentration. She did the same on my left wrist and took my blood pressure. It was 110 over 70.

I looked blank so she added, "That's very good."

I looked around the room and noticed a framed photo of a man in orange robes and a sculpture that looked like a small animal skull on her bookcase. I was idly reading her diplomas when she said, "OK, I need to review this information, so now is a good time if you have to get some water or use the restroom."

Victoria and I headed out to the hallway, and I realized how tense I was. "Wow, it's awful." I told Victoria, "Even though Dr. Desai is nice, I'm really afraid of doctors now."

"That makes sense. You had a pretty bad experience."

"I know, right?" I said. "MS is a pretty difficult diagnosis, isn't it? Mostly a diagnosis of last resort?"

"It's supposed to be a diagnosis of exclusion," she said. "You have to exclude everything else."

Back in the office, Victoria and I sat quietly while Dr. Desai finished making notes. "OK, I'm going to explain it to you in both Western and Eastern traditions."

"Do you believe a body can heal?"

"Yes," she said. "Do I think I can help people get closer to health? Yes. Now if you were in a wheelchair, I'm not saying I could get you up and walking again. I don't know..."

Again I cut her off. "It's a philosophical question. After Dr. Silver, I promised myself I wouldn't see another doctor without asking if we were in alignment. I believe the body wants to be in balance and in health so we need to figure out what's in the way of that. Do you believe that?"

She looked slightly confused, maybe a little annoyed (I don't blame her given all my interruptions), but she agreed. "Yes, I believe that. I come from a different perspective. It's unlike other doctors."

I nodded.

"Now," she smiled, "I'm going to explain it to you in both Western and Eastern traditions. From the Eastern medical perspective, your *vata* is out of balance," Dr. Desai said. "Your constitution is *vata-kapha*..."

And, again, I cut her off. (I've got to stop doing this.) "Really?" I ask, my voice rising eagerly. I'd learned the basics of Ayurveda from Deepak Chopra's book. I'd read about *vata*, *pitta* and *kapha*, the three *doshas*, or mind-body personalities in Sanskrit. All of us are born with a specific combination of the three, and according to Ayurveda, keeping them in balance is the key to good health.

I knew I was *vata*. Everything I'd read about it sounded like me: woven from the elements of air and space, *vata* types tend to be lean and long limbed. They're energetic and agile. They are comfortable with and even eager for change, they live in constant motion, and they crave creativity over security in their work.

All of it was me: I have trouble finding shirts with long-enough sleeves and I couldn't gain weight if my life depended on it. I'm a writer with little financial security and endless amounts of frequent-flier miles. And there's that problem of forwarding addresses: I've lived in ten cities in six states since I left Detroit as a seventeen-year-old.

After *vata*, I figured I was *pitta*, the element of fire that makes people intense, opinionated and often outspoken. That sounded like me too, although I really wanted to be *kapha*. When I read *Perfect Health*, I really, truly yearned to be that solid and sensible combination of earth and water. *Kapha* types are healthy, sturdy and reliable. If they RSVP, they show up. They don't miss your wedding because they can't get a flight out of Indonesia. *Kapha* types have tremendous endurance, and physically, they're the non-*vata*. They gain weight when they eat too much or forget to exercise, and they never feel like a good wind could send them off course.

I often feel like one good gust and I'm outta here. I've never been confused for sturdy. And for the last year, I'm the one who didn't believe I was healthy. After the whole Dr. Silver fiasco, I forgot that for the first forty-two years of life, I ran marathons at will and never stayed in a hospital, never suffered illness more intense than a cold, and never broke a bone despite all my adventures.

"Yes," Dr. Desai continued, "it's your *kapha* that kept you healthy most of your life. It makes you strong physically. *Kapha* types are good at endurance sports. It gives you good physical and emotional endurance."

At this point, I was so happy I could hardly think and yet, it was about to get better.

"You're not that unhealthy," she said. "You're not that far from optimal health."

And with that, I went from happy to elated. I was intensely relieved to know there was a doctor nearby who understood me and all my intertwined systems and saw them as close to optimal health. I was so relieved that I could barely concentrate on what Dr. Desai was saying as she started to explain those systems. She started talking about subcategories of *doshas* and the pulses she checked and what it all meant. "Your *prana*, *tejas* and *ojas* are all normal," she said. These are the vital essences that control mind-body function.

That sounded good. The next level down, the seven bodily tissues, showed something less good. Basically, Dr. Desai said, my kidney and adrenal pulses were weak, and there was something going on in my small intestine. She flipped back through some of the pages I sent and asked about chelation.

I explained what I understood from Dr. Duncan, the woman I saw in the spring who had tested me for metal toxicity—that the heavy metals in my system were causing the tingling and I needed to take a chelating agent to remove them.

"That's one theory," Dr. Desai said. "Here's what I believe happened. Before the tingling started, you went to Mexico and got some sort of stomach bug. That's why your stomach hurt. Western medicine is not equipped to read the most subtle changes, so your doctors said it was nothing.

"Because of what was going on in your intestine, you were unable to absorb nutrients from your food and you developed an extreme B12 deficiency," Dr. Desai continued. "The first symptom of a B12 deficiency is tingling in the fingers and toes. You started feeling better because you started supplementing your diet with vitamins. Then you started doing chelation, which takes everything out of your system, and you started feeling bad again."

And then, in much kinder language, she basically said my diet stunk. I thought it was überhealthy. I followed the food rules set out by Michael Pollan: real food, mostly plants and not too much of any one thing in particular—at least I thought. What could be better than that?

Meat and chicken would be. Both are good sources of vitamin B12, and I rarely ate either. When Dr. Desai went through my diet, she pointed out that I rarely ate any protein at all—not a good strategy for healing.

She sent me home with a few herbal formulas to get my gut back in order. She also gave very clear—even illustrated—directions to eat balanced meals. She drew a circle broken into four quadrants, with letters in each—P, C, F, V. "At every meal, you must eat protein, carbs (100 percent whole grain or a starchy vegetable), fat and a cooked vegetable."

The cooking part, she said, was critical. I didn't have the intestinal fortitude to break down raw plants.

*Cool*, I thought. *I cooked in restaurants. I'm happy to cook all my food, forgo raw carrots if that means no more weirdness in my feet, no more fear of MS and no more thoughts of Dr. Silver and his proposed plan of weekly injections.*

I thanked Dr. Desai and practically floated out of her office. Six inches of snow had fallen while I was inside. It was the light, airy, fluffy kind, so I happily brushed it off my car and climbed in.

I drove a few minutes and merged onto the freeway, where loads of cars stood motionless pointing toward Denver. I called Lisa, who turned me on to the Department of Transportation website. I thought she might be at her desk so I asked her to take a look for me.

"Sure," she said, and laughed out loud. "I'm sorry, I've just never seen anything like this. It says the speed on US 36 is zero. You may never get home."

"Oh, well," I said, "I don't care. I don't have MS. I just have to cook my vegetables. And eat more protein."

"That's great, Jo," Lisa said. She didn't really need to hear it from Dr. Desai. She already believed it was a misdiagnosis. She had believed it was BS since I told her about the first four doctors who said it wasn't MS.

I was the only one who had kept a constant, if low-level, fear going.

As I sat in traffic, then rolled ten feet forward and stopped again, I wondered why. Was low-level fear the inevitable by-product of a full-blown panic, just a lingering effect of that initial shock? Would it go away in time? Or was something still unresolved?

As the snow fell and I inched my way home, rolling forward and stopping, rolling and stopping, I was so happy and excited that I couldn't stay right where I was. I decided I needed one last thing to cap this whole year of diagnosis-induced insanity. I decided to call Dr. Deborah Lee, a respected and well-known neurologist whom Dr. Duncan (the heavy metal expert) had suggested I call. I didn't want another opinion. Dr. Lee billed herself as a "holistic neurologist," so I thought her opinion would be the same as Drs. Martin, Darmal, and Desai: not MS. And while I trusted each of them, none was an apples-to-apples comparison with Silver. And none had given me something official and formal that I could submit to my insurance company to refute Silver's comments. As long as Silver's opinion sat heavy on my medical records, I could never get another insurance plan, not at a rate I could afford. At the time, a preexisting condition was enough to deny a person insurance or charge her exorbitant rates, and in the insurance gatekeeper's minds, I had a dreaded pre-existing condition.

As I slowly rolled home, I relaxed because not only could I clear this mess from my record, I could clear it from my mind. Dr. Desai looked at all the evidence and linked it in a way that made sense of all the twists and turns: the stomachache that preceded the tingling, the tingling itself and the way it left my hands and later came back in my toes.

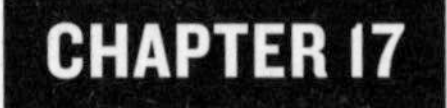

# PACKING ICE IN YOUR POCKETS

I called Dr. Lee and made an appointment for February 1—three days before I was set to fly to Kenya to travel with a friend and go on safari with Bruce.

He'd been traveling back and forth to Kenya for ten or twelve months, working to put together a complicated business deal that somehow involved a gold mine, German geologists and the Turkana people of northern Kenya. About once a month, maybe more, he'd fly to Nairobi, board a smaller plane and continue to a spot near the Ugandan border, where he would then camp in the bush, scope out the potential mining operation and negotiate with tribesmen, Kenyan officials and the Germans. For a businessman who had worked on mining projects all over the globe for years, I could tell he was exceptionally happy about this one, almost gleeful. The deal was going to be so big that Bruce had his entire team on it, and to my surprise, he even found a spot for me. "I'll tell you what," he had said one day in the fall. "We're going to need someone to publicize this. I'd like to hire you to do corporate communications, and as a member of our team, your airfare and expenses will be covered."

I had needed precisely zero seconds to squeal, "*Yes*! Absolutely,

I'd love to. Oh my God, this so great. I can't wait. Thank you, thank you!"

"You're welcome," he said. "It's going to be great. I'm really glad you'll be a part of it."

And a few seconds later, I squealed again, "Oh my God, this is going to be amazing. I'll go with you to Africa and we'll see lions and tigers and elephants."

"I don't think you'll see tigers," Bruce said. "They don't have 'em in Kenya. Lions for sure, and giraffes, elephants too, but no tigers. I'm sorry, honey, is that a deal breaker for you?"

"No, definitely not." And we both laughed.

We had already finalized the dates when we were together over Christmas, long before I'd seen Dr. Desai. And then, with amazing serendipity, when I was back in Denver in January and still squealing about my impending African adventure, a woman I knew from the yoga studio said she too was going to Kenya in February. She had traveled there after college and was going back to visit members of the Samburu tribe she'd befriended then.

"The Samburu live right near the Turkana. Why don't you come with me?" she'd asked. And again, I took precisely zero seconds to say, "Absolutely, I'd love to." I figured, what were the chances that two people I knew from entirely different places, who were completely unconnected to one another, were both going to the same remote region of northwest Kenya at the exact same time? And both invited me to travel with them? I had to say yes.

Then, in early January, when I called Dr. Lee, it didn't occur to me that seeing a neurologist—holistic or otherwise—three days before an international flight was something I'd tried before.

In the weeks leading up to the two events, I started feeling anxious about the trip. I started calling Bruce almost daily to ask about it, and although I didn't know it, I wasn't the only one. When he wasn't on the phone with me, the geologists and the Kenyans he was negotiating with were calling to pepper him with questions, problems and demands, until one day, the entire deal blew apart. No gold, no life-changing project and no payoff for the year of his life and the dollars already invested.

I tried to console him, but he didn't want to talk too much about the deal, so I asked if he still wanted to make a vacation out of it and go on safari with me.

"Uh, yeah, I think I can make that work. Just take a phone with you when you're with your friend so I can reach you if I can't make it."

The real appeal of Africa was spending time with Bruce. The first few weeks, with a woman I barely knew and a nomadic, goat-herding tribe—that sounded like an exciting adventure and only the lead-in to working with and vacationing with Bruce. And now he was saying he may call during the first part of the trip to cancel the second and better part of it. *Shoot.* And I'd be in some undisclosed location surrounded by goats. Cell service seemed unlikely. Disaster seemed probable.

And swiftly, without the safety and security I felt about traveling with Bruce, I started feeling less safe and secure about other events happening in the same time frame. It was as if one plan falling apart proved that another, unrelated plan could unravel too. I started worrying about seeing another neurologist and what she might say.

The morning of my appointment with Dr. Lee, I woke up wishing for a blizzard to close all the roads. When I got out of bed and took Riley for a walk, there was no snow in sight. I drove into the suburbs and took a seat in the waiting room.

When Dr. Lee stuck her head in to say she'd be with me in a minute, I immediately thought, *That's what the tooth fairy would look like, if there were a tooth fairy.* She was tiny—maybe five feet tall and a hundred pounds. She wore a flowy purple skirt with flowers on it, a small cardigan and kitten-heeled black suede boots. Her towhead blond hair was shoulder length and nearly translucent around her small pale white face.

I checked the books on her bookshelf, flipping through some until Dr. Lee returned. She introduced herself and said she was a neurologist who had gone back to school to study biochemistry. She said this was very difficult, starting all over again in school, after she was already a neurologist, but she felt it was important to understand the impact of nutrition on neurology.

Dr. Lee started flipping through the mess of paperwork that I had filled out and mailed in earlier. I handed her the CD with the MRIs on it—the same one I had shared with Dr. Martin in Vancouver and Dr. Darmal in California.

"Thanks," she said, putting the CD on her desk and flipping to the health privacy pages. "Where do you want me to send my report and the results of this exam?"

"It's on the form, isn't it?" I asked. "Just send everything to me."

"You don't want me to send it to your insurance? Or to Dr. Duncan?"

Dr. Duncan originally gave me Dr. Lee's name, but I hadn't seen Dr. Duncan since I stopped doing the chelation. "That depends," I said. "If you're going to say I don't have MS, send it far and wide. If you're going to say I do, then send it to me and only to me."

"It was Dr. Duncan who referred you, right? Do you want me to send it to her?"

"No, just send it to me, like I wrote on the form."

And from there, she went through the rest of the pile page by page asking me what I ate, how I slept, if I'd ever been in a car accident or fallen on my head. Her interview was a combination of

Dr. Martin, Dr. Desai and therapy. She asked about the house where I grew up, about my mom, dad and sister. She asked if we all got along and if my parents were still together.

Dr. Lee asked about the trip to Ecuador—the same one Martin asked about where I grew loopy at altitude. She asked what else happened after the trip, so I told her not much, other than when I got back to New York, I couldn't eat. "I mean I could eat," I said, "but if I did, I had to run for the bathroom."

"Diarrhea?" she asked.

"Yeah," I said. "I lost a dozen pounds and when I called my doctor at the time, she wrote a prescription for Cipro. Gave it to me over the phone. I didn't even see her. But the Cipro seemed to kill whatever it was."

"How long did you take it?"

"Three days, I think."

Dr. Lee frowned and looked back at the pages.

"Does Cipro mean something?" I asked. She explained that it kills everything in a gut—not just the bad bugs but all the good ones too. It's like napalm. If a person takes Cipro without taking probiotics, it leaves the intestinal tract in rough shape—no good bacteria to digest food or to fight off incoming bad bacteria.

Dr. Lee asked more questions about my life, my family and my health. She asked about every other doctor I had seen, what they said and what I thought about them. The interview portion of this appointment went on for a while—ninety minutes or more—and I felt like I was auditioning for a part or sitting in a job interview. Or presenting my case in court.

Even though I felt great physically and had no complaints, I felt like the burden of proof was on me. I felt like I had a felony on my record that needed to be expunged, that I had no power in the process, and that the tooth fairy was judge and jury. At least Dr. Lee seemed a kinder judge and jury than Silver. I was grateful for that. And I was relaxing, starting to trust her, and to trust that this would work out as planned—that she would give me proof that Silver was wrong that I could submit to my insurance. And then, after this long year, I could say good-bye to the HMO's doctors who'd let me down, apply for new insurance and with no preexisting condition, join some other plan and be done with the whole scary affair. Graduation day. That was the plan.

"You know," she said, putting all the paperwork back together in a pile. "I think your intestinal tract has always been your weak link. When you were a kid, you might not have realized how much stress was in your house, but your GI tract did."

"Yeah," I said, "Dr. Desai thought it was an intestinal thing too."

I didn't mention that Dr. Desai said I was close to optimal health. I just thought it. And became more confident that the tooth fairy would confirm it.

"So you don't think it's MS?"

"C'mon, I'll show you into the exam room."

She showed me across the hall to a tiny room, with the same cold white paper covering the exam table. She handed me a paper dress and a blanket. "In case you get cold," she said. "I'll be right back."

I took off my clothes and put them on the chair. I put my arms through the paper gown so it was open in back, wrapped the blanket around me and took a seat on the table, swinging my feet over the edge. And then I waited. And waited some more. There was no bookshelf in the exam room, so I looked at the ceiling, then looked at the floor and wondered which of the drunk-driving tests she would ask me to do and why I had to be nearly naked when I did them. Drunks weren't naked when they took the tests, not usually anyway. And if she was going to look in my ears and eyes, she'd see the same thing if I were wearing pants.

After what seemed an unreasonably long time, Dr. Lee knocked and entered the room. She took out a small metallic case that held a pointed flashlight to look in my ears. She looked in one, then walked around and moved my hair to look in the other. Even though she was right next to me, touching me, looking in my ear, she was somehow distant and different.

She looked the same—small, blond with a purple skirt—and yet I felt like I'd never met her before. The woman who asked questions and listened patiently to my answers was now cold and hard, like the small metal case she placed beside me. The tooth fairy was gone, replaced by something more robotic.

"OK, now I'll listen to your lungs," she said.

The energy in the room had changed. The energy between us had changed. So much that I had to comment.

"We were having such a nice open-ended conversation and now it's like you're a doctor again, a doctor on a mission," I said.

Dr. Lee didn't say anything and put the cold metal on my back and then on my chest. Then she pulled out a little white card with the familiar letters: L E F O D P T C.

As I went to read them, I realized my shoulders were floating up near my ears. I was growing tense and breathing short, shallow breaths. "It's only an eye exam," I said out loud. "There are no wrong answers."

I was audibly talking myself down from the ledge, and Dr. Lee said nothing. She waited for me to read, checked my peripheral vision and had me follow her pen with my eyes as she moved it right to left.

"Good," she said and took out the rubber triangle hammer and knocked just below my left knee.

"You're reflexes are brisk," she said.

My reflexes have always been called brisk. When I was a kid, the doctor always commented on my reflexes. Every time, he'd say, "Oooh, better stand back on these." I figured he said it to all his patients.

Dr. Lee put the hammer back in its slot and took a cold tuning fork out of the case. She struck it and held it to my big toe. "Tell me when it stops vibrating."

After a moment when the thing settled down, I said, "Now." She struck the thing again and placed the cold metal on one cold toe and then another and another. "Now," "now," and "now," I said.

Dr. Lee put her tools away and closed the case. "Stand up for me."

I did.

"Let's have you walk heel to toe, forward."

"Dr. Silver had me do that backward," I said.

"I've never asked anyone to do that backward," she laughed, almost sneering at how silly his test was. "That's like asking someone to fall over." That made me relax a little bit. And after I finished going forward, she said, "OK, stand up on your toes. Balance on the balls of your feet."

I did that too. No problem.

"Now, just balance on your right foot, up on your toes."

"Up like this?" I asked as I lifted my left foot and stayed on the ball of my right until she said, "OK, and now the left foot."

I put my left foot down, lifted my right foot behind me and raised up onto the ball of my left foot. And soon I got wobbly.

Dr. Lee frowned. And looked down.

"OK," she said. "Get dressed and I'll meet you back in the office."

I put on my clothes and pulled my snugly Ugg boots onto my now-freezing-cold toes and went back across the hall to her office.

Dr. Lee was sitting behind her desk, facing the table against the wall with her back to me. Before I even sat down, she turned in her chair to face me and handed me a box of Kleenex. "Here, have a seat," she said, motioning to the chair beside her, where we could both see the screen of her laptop.

"I want you to focus on how resilient and redundant the human neurological system is," she started.

Now I understood why the energy had changed between the interview and the exam. I understood why I waited so long in the exam room. While I changed and waited, she had looked at the MRI.

"Oh, fuck," I said. "Let's cut to the chase here. You think I have MS, don't you?"

"Well," she said, "this is a classic MS MRI. Sit down, let me show you what we're looking at."

She started with a contrast image of my cervical spine, where she pointed out how the vertebrae in my neck were small and close together. "You have degenerative disc disease," she said evenly—as if this were no big deal and not a completely new disease for me, one that every other expert failed to mention. She didn't linger on that and pointed out the white spots in the spinal cord itself. "Look, here's one, two," pointing at the screen with her pen. "Three, four, five, six...It's quite a bit of inflammation."

Dr. Lee explained that the image we were looking at was a slice of my spinal cord. She took me through the images of my brain too, slice after slice, and pointed out a pair of white spots there too.

I said, "All right, so there are lesions. How do we make them go away?"

She smiled and didn't answer.

"Well, do lesions come and go?" I asked.

"Yeah, they do go away," she said and drifted off, as if this weren't a thought worth finishing.

Anxiety was rising in my chest. My feet were sweating in their ugly Ugg boots.

"So if you MRI'ed a hundred people at random," I asked, "I mean, if you pulled a hundred people out of the parking lot at Safeway and MRI'ed their heads, how many of them would have lesions?"

"There are some asymptomatic lesions," she said, "and we can talk about that later."

But we didn't talk about that. Not then and not later. Instead of following that train of thought, instead of answering my question, she turned to me and said, "If you need to cry or yell, go ahead. You can."

And at that moment, I did need to cry. And not just because I suddenly was back to square one, thinking I was going to die of MS. That was only part of it. I feared the disease, but mostly I started bawling because I couldn't hold it back anymore. I was frustrated from not being heard, not having my questions answered, and being told I was damaged.

But I also suddenly didn't have it in me to say one more time, "What the hell? What about those hundred people at Safeway? What about the asymptomatic lesions? What about my GI tract being the weak link? Or the nutritional deficiencies or trauma or anything any of the other doctors said? Or what about what *you* said before you looked at the stupid MRI?"

Exhausted from what seemed a lifetime of trying to convince someone that I was fine and healthy and important enough to be heard, I could only sob.

Dr. Lee waited. And the more I cried, the more patiently she waited. Until she finally said, "Dr. Silver likely didn't return your calls or answer your emails because he hasn't done his own work, he hasn't learned to sit with his own pain so he wasn't comfortable sitting with yours. Few doctors do the work."

As my breathing slowly returned to normal, Dr. Lee told me she was a Buddhist, that she had a great teacher, that she was trained to deal with what is.

I listened. I liked talking about Buddhist philosophy.

"What Dr. Silver told you about chicken pox, that doesn't make sense," Dr. Lee said, back in her tooth fairy voice. "I think you have leaky gut syndrome, which means food stays in your digestive tract too long without getting broken down."

When food doesn't get broken down, she explained, pieces that are too big eventually slip through the intestinal wall into the bloodstream and wreak havoc. She said my body couldn't recognize these larger particles as self, so my immune system attacked them as invaders. The immune system created an inflammatory response—which is its job—but ultimately the immune system went too far and crossed the blood-brain barrier into my central nervous system.

This scenario sounded plausible and seemed to match Dr. Desai's theory. Except Dr. Lee wasn't going to say, "You're not far from optimal health."

She suggested I change my diet. "I'm sure Dr. Desai has talked to you about that," she said. "And you should go on interferon drugs."

Immediately, reflexively, I started crying again.

When I could talk, I said, "Wait a minute, I've only ever had the tingling in my fingertips and the weird sensation in my feet. You didn't find anything in the exam so couldn't the tingling have been an ergonomic thing? I was sitting at a laptop all day with my arms like this," I rounded my back and held my hands on some imaginary Barbie laptop, "and that tingling went away when I started stretching, taking vitamins and got a new keyboard."

"I think the tingling in your fingers could have been ergonomic, but the toes, that's MS," she said.

I stared in silence, unclear how to untangle or articulate my disbelief.

"I'm not an MS expert," she said. "There are three at the university hospital."

She spun around back to her laptop, with her back to me, and looked at the hospital's website. She went through each doctor, told me that each was very brilliant and described their personalities.

"I don't want to take interferons," I said. "Silver suggested them too and when I looked into them, they all sounded awful."

"I would take them," she said. "I would if I were you."

She had no trouble telling me what she would do in my condition, mostly because she was not in my condition, which at the moment was exhausted, frustrated, scared and—on top of all that—feeling physically strong and flexible. The only interesting thing she discovered during the physical exam was that I could balance longer on my right toe than left. I can throw a ball farther with my right arm too, but who cares? No one would argue that's a sign of MS.

"I leave for Borneo next week," Dr. Lee said. "We can reconvene when I return. Oh, wait you said you're leaving the country too. Are you going to Kenya?"

I nodded. "On Monday."

"Heat is not great for MS patients," Dr. Lee said, frowning. And just like Silver, she went into certainty mode, talking about MS patients as if she had no doubt that I was one. "I know you can't stay out of the heat there but try to manage it. Put ice in your pockets to stay cool."

"I'm traveling with a nomadic goat-herding tribe," I said. "No electricity and no running water. Ice will be difficult."

This tooth fairy was persistent. "Go to Costco or someplace and get a battery-operated fan to keep with you."

I looked at her like she was from Pluto. She had traveled off to this strange planet where a year of feeling OK and a perfect physical exam matters less than one MRI taken at one moment in time one year ago. Even though her certainty scared me, I had come too far over this past year to let someone else bully me into believing this diagnosis on their word alone. At the same time, I still wanted to understand what she was saying.

"Hang on," I said. "What do you mean the heat is bad for people with MS?"

And now Dr. Lee looked at me like I was speaking another language.

"I mean," I continued, "if you're talking about discomfort, I can live with discomfort. Or are you talking about something else?"

"Well," she said, and wrinkled her nose like something smelled. "The heat can cause problems. It can exacerbate symptoms or cause new ones."

Hot tubs, in fact, used to be the primary means of diagnosis. Prior to the advent of MRI machines, doctors tossed patients in a hot tub. If their symptoms grew worse, the diagnosis was MS.

"You'll probably be OK," she said. "But find a battery-operated fan."

CHAPTER 18

# THE BABOONS ARE BRAWLING

Lisa picked me up around six for dinner. My eyes were puffy and red, and she wasn't surprised. Earlier, on the phone, I'd already started crying.

"This was supposed to be like my graduation dinner," I said, continuing where we left off. Normally, I'd try to stop myself but Lisa and I met in kindergarten. There's comfort and safety in an old friendship, and license to be a little kid. "The doctor was supposed to clear me of this whole nightmare and now, I don't know, I mean, she thinks I have MS and that going to Africa could make it worse."

Lisa's a thoughtful listener. I told her that Dr. Lee and I talked for two hours and that the conversation seemed to go well. I told Lisa about the physical exam and that nothing was unusual except that I could balance longer on one foot than the other.

"Standing up on the ball of your foot?" Lisa asked. "I probably couldn't pass that test either." A triathlete who mountain bikes rough terrain all summer and skis Colorado backcountry all winter, Lisa's the best athlete I know. One time, careening down a two-lane highway on a road bike near Durango, she saw a small blur running into her path. As she got closer, she realized it was a bear that she couldn't avoid. She careened off his shoulder, rode out the skid and continued on, leaving a stunned bear to scramble back into the woods while she peddled home. If Lisa can't do something, I figure it can't be done.

"The whole vibe changed when Dr. Lee came into the exam room," I said. "She'd looked at the MRI and then everything was different. The open-ended questions were gone and she was on a quest for evidence of MS.

"She told me to take the drugs," I said.

"You know," Lisa said as she drove toward our favorite divey Thai restaurant. "It doesn't surprise me that two doctors with the same training would analyze the same data in the same way."

"Yeah?" I said, eager to hear more on this line of thought.

"They're both trained to read an MRI the same way, and you showed her the same MRI," Lisa said. "She's going to see the same thing he did. I'm not sure you have any more information now than you had before."

"Huh," I said, unable to say anymore while that sunk in. We drove in silence, parked and found a table in the tiny joint. We ordered spicier food than I'd have ordered on my own and got back to talking about my day.

"I'm just feeling so shitty about the whole thing," I said. "I mean why did I set up another neurology appointment just days before another big trip? How stupid was that?"

"It wasn't stupid," Lisa said. "You're going to take off Monday and have an amazing time and forget all about this."

"I don't know, Dr. Lee said the heat could make things worse."

"If you had MS, that may be true," Lisa said. "But there are no real signs of it, right? You're not feeling bad now, are you? What do think will get worse? And you've been to Mexico a half dozen times since the first dude told you the MRI meant MS and nothing happened on any of those trips."

"You're right. I have been in the heat a bunch."

In addition to being a skilled outdoor athlete, Lisa's a world-class adventurer—she served in the Peace Corps in Guatemala; biked alone through Vietnam, Cambodia and Laos; and toured Central America, South America and Europe. For an entire year in her twenties, she was a full-time traveler. She bought an around-the-world airline ticket and explored, day after day, month after month, with no agenda other than to enjoy and experience the world.

I knew what she would do if she were me: go to Africa.

No question, Lisa would get on a plane without a second thought. She's a good friend. She's fearless. I'd always wanted to be like her. I decided it was now time to do so.

The next morning, I woke up, walked my dog, stretched and sat down to meditate. When I finished, I brought my hands together in prayer and made a mental list of all the things that felt like a blessing. "I'm grateful for this light, this love, this life, this mind, this body, all the healing I've done, all the teachings and all my teachers, in this and every present moment."

Lisa definitely ranked high on the list of teachers. Bruce too.

As I made breakfast, I gave him a call and left a message. He emailed a few hours later to say he was sorry to hear the appointment didn't go well and that he had more bad news. He couldn't make it to Nairobi. He wasn't feeling well and didn't have it in him to fly that far.

I wanted to cry. I wasn't surprised, but I was crushed.

I ate breakfast; pulled on a jacket, hat and gloves; and rounded up Riley for her second walk of the still-new day. We got as far as the Platte River Trail, about fifteen minutes away, when I wanted to cry again. I contemplated calling Lisa but stopped myself. She had done her share of emotional heavy lifting with me the night before.

I walked a little while longer and called my dad.

"OK," he said. "Tell me what happened."

I told him about the appointment and Lisa's idea about doctors with the same training reaching the same conclusion.

"I think she's right. You've been feeling really good and what you did learn yesterday is that on a physical exam, there were no signs of MS," my dad said. "Focus on that."

"So I should go, right Dad?"

He didn't hesitate and, for a man who considers riding in a compact car "roughing it," he was overwhelmingly in favor of Africa.

"Go," he said. "Go and enjoy yourself and in the fullness of time, a more accurate diagnosis will be found."

I love my dad.

I spent the rest of the day packing the usual suspects—shorts, T-shirts and sunblock—into a backpack alongside a water purifier and big bags of nuts, seeds and protein bars, just in case there wasn't much to eat or anything safe to drink.

Monday afternoon, I boarded a flight from Denver to Heathrow, where I drank tea in a restaurant and wrote notes in my journal. I wrote about the doctor's appointment and my conversation with Lisa. And about the nonconversation with Bruce. Ultimately, though, I wrote about me and what my body was saying. "I believe my body can heal," I wrote. I still had a nagging feeling that something wasn't quite right and a deep-seated belief that it didn't have to be permanent.

Hours later, I boarded a flight to Nairobi.

Michelle, my yoga friend, had flown in a few days earlier, so she and her Samburu buddy, Lepikayo, picked me up at the airport. Five nine, he was stocky and dressed like an American in long, baggy jean shorts, a Colorado State University T-shirt and a long chain with a gold ram's head hanging around his neck. His skin was reddish brown, not the blue black I'd expected. His teeth where shiny and white, and he had a gap-toothed smile on the lower jaw.

Lepikayo said hello and threw my luggage in the back of the car. We pulled out of the airport, drove through Nairobi traffic and smog, and headed north for seven sweaty hours over emptier and emptier, bumpier and bumpier, roads. In the late afternoon, we arrived at Samburu National Reserve, home to Elsa and her cubs from *Born Free*.

Inside the park, we immediately saw a family of elephants. Enormous and majestic, they stood in clumps—two over there, three over there, and another four or five a bit further behind. All standing in the big, open space, bathed in the late afternoon light, the elephants somehow made my jet lag disappear. Wide awake, I pressed my nose to the window like a little kid.

"There's a baby," Lepikayo yelled and pointed the forty-year-old Range Rover in that direction. As we got closer to the biggest clump of elephants, we could see a little one that stood no taller than the other ones' armpits. "It can't be more than a couple of days old," Lepikayo said, putting the car in park.

As we sat staring and oohing and aahing, the elephants started lumbering toward us. Swinging their trunks and slogging their mighty feet forward one at a time, they moved with deceptive speed. Quickly, they were close enough that we could see their eyes and the detailed outline of their ears.

Several of the animals moved between us and the little one. The biggest elephant covered the most ground, coming from way back, behind the pack, a hundred yards away to plant himself within forty feet of us. He stopped and stared and spread his big ears out to either side as if to say, "I'm even bigger than you think. Back up."

We snapped a few photos and decided to leave the family in peace. We turned around and continued through the open space, with the sun moving lower in the sky to our left. We saw a trio of giraffes eating from the tops of the trees, not ten feet from our window, and a handful of zebras grazing in the tall grass. We watched antelopes and impalas bounding about, and we saw one other car, a newer, flashier Range Rover with white faces and fancy cameras poking out of the popped top.

Eventually, as the light grew dim, we started the search for our campsite. The park had moved it since the last time Lepikayo visited, so the search took some doing. We arrived in the dark, and while Lepikayo negotiated with the guard, I stood near the car with my head tossed back, staring at the sky. It was as dark a sky as I'd ever seen, with more stars than I'd ever seen anywhere. In northern Michigan, where there's next to no light pollution, I'd seen brilliant displays of sparkling lights, but this African night was another order of magnitude.

Millions and millions of shiny, twinkling white spots splattered across the dark sky, held tight by the frothy white stripe of the Milky Way. It was amazing and breathtaking, and as I inhaled the scene, I knew I was about to crash. It had been fifty hours since I'd boarded the flight in Denver. My T-shirt was ripe, and I couldn't tell if I was hungry. I didn't feel exhausted—way past that—and I knew I was done for the day.

The campsite consisted of six tall, green A-frame tents built on wooden platforms. They were set up around a kitchen area with several long tables under a tarp. The outhouse was ten yards away, and we met the night watchman who walked the perimeter with a shotgun each night. If animals came into camp, he was prepared to shoot the sky to scare them away.

Inside the tent, I was grateful to see cots already made up with scratchy white sheets. I searched my bag for my head lamp, a toothbrush and my bright green sleeping-bag liner. I slid the thing between the sheets, crawled in and fell asleep almost instantly.

Hours later, I woke to big, thundering noises. *Thump, thump, crash, crash, thump.* The ruckus sounded like it was just beyond the canvas wall. I wanted to lift the window flap to see what was going on, and at the same time, I wanted to stay very still. Whatever it was didn't sound dangerous, just really, really big, and maybe a little uncoordinated.

*Thump. Thump. Crash. Thump. Crash.*

"Are you guys awake?" I asked so quietly that my words were almost inaudible.

"Yes" came back equally small.

"What do we do?"

"Nothing."

I lay still, listening to thumping and branches breaking until sleep took over.

In the morning, I bounded out of bed at six to full daylight. I walked around the tent to see what had happened and saw broken branches, scuffs in the dirt and enormous circles, one the size of a hubcap just six inches from the tent wall. While I was staring at it, trying to make sense of it, Lepikayo came around. "An elephant footprint, probably a baby," he said and walked away.

If I had stuck my arm out the tent window, I would have touched elephant. Wild.

After breakfast, we climbed into the dusty green Rover and drove through the park looking for animals. We saw giraffes, elephants and gazelles. We saw one lion walking alone along a ridge, slowly, sweetly, as if she were enjoying herself and the view. We followed along, thirty feet behind her. She knew we were there and didn't care, just kept doing a model-like strut, swinging her hips and tail, moving slowly and purposefully with her head held high until she found her spot and sat herself down like royalty.

Midmorning, we drove to the Samburu Game Lodge, a luxurious palace of a hotel where I imagine Ernest Hemingway would have stayed. Thatched roofs stood tall over the long wooden bar, and the sprawling deck offered a view of the mostly dry Ewaso Nyiro River. Lazy ceiling fans barely moved the hot, heavy air. Tables and chairs sat empty. Monkeys ran along the railing and onto the bar, where they helped themselves to sugar packets until the waiters shooed them away with shouts and slingshots.

Michelle, Lepikayo and I took a seat on a plush sofa and ordered three fruit juices. The waiter left and sometime later returned with tall glasses, filled with a sweet orange liquid and one ice cube floating in each. We chatted about nothing much and watched the monkeys and the men with slingshots until we were ready to head back to our campsite in search of lunch or a nap. On the way out, I stopped at the front desk—another expansive stretch of carved wood under the shade of the thatched roof. On the wall behind the desk, I saw a thermometer: 120 degrees, in the shade. In. The. Shade. If heat was going to hurt me, this counted as heat. And I felt great.

That night, again, I woke in the dark to a new, more frenetic symphony of crazy crashing sounds. As I lay motionless, listening to screeches and snaps and collapses, I thought it sounded like a barroom brawl, the kind on TV where everyone gets pulled in: men breaking chairs over one another's backs, women screaming and glass shattering. The brawling continued unabated, neither growing louder nor calming down, until sleep took over again.

In the morning I asked Lepikayo about it. "Baboons," he said. "They were fighting in the trees."

On day three, we awoke at four in the morning, got in the car and left the park, pointed for more remote and rougher terrain. We drove and drove—or more accurately, Lepikayo wrestled the vehicle over rocky roads that became sandy paths with deep potholes and brutally bumpy stretches. We saw ostriches running in packs and little kids walking alone. We weathered the obscene heat and the gasoline fumes coming off the engine into the workhorse of a car.

Late in the afternoon, when we were so dusty and sweaty that it was impossible to tell the real color of our skin, we descended a small slope to a dry riverbed, where two little kids, a girl and a boy not more than seven, stood surrounded by hundreds of black-and-white goats. Lepikayo rolled down his window and shouted a burst of syllables in Samburu. The kids came running over. They each had the same gap-toothed smile as Lepikayo. "These are my brother's kids," he said, "and his goats."

After a brief conversation, Lepikayo said good-bye and continued driving along the center of the wide, flat riverbed that hadn't seen water in years. The drought was in its third year.

We came to a bend in the river where Lepikayo had set up a camp for us. He'd built six traditional Samburu homes—or had women in his tribe build them from sticks woven together with reeds. Each had about the same footprint as a twin bed. The roofs, made of smaller twigs, were about four feet high. I could duck inside and sit cross-legged if I wanted. No standing though. Traditionally, an entire family, parents and kids and all, would sleep inside one of these babies. I was lucky—or maybe unlucky—and had my own.

The camp sat near a watering hole dug deep into the scorched earth. Every morning, young boys would come with their goats or camels or donkeys. One boy would drop down into the hole, fill a bucket with water and hand it to another boy, who would dump it into a trough to water the animals. The boys would chant an easy rhythm and the animals would bray and snort and slosh.

Lepikayo and his friends, five Samburu men, sat in the shade between our huts, playing a game with pebbles and a small wooden board. As I sat and watched them one day, I couldn't make heads or tails of the game, but I realized they all had the same smile as Lepikayo and his brother's kids. All of them had a gap between their bottom front teeth.

Later, I asked Michelle about this, and she explained it was a tribal custom that began when babies suffered lockjaw from the tetanus bacteria. Saddened by watching baby after baby die, the tribal elders decided to remove front teeth as a prophylactic. The kids would live with a gap-toothed smile, but they could get food and medicine even if they couldn't open their mouths.

Tetanus is no longer a baby killer in most parts of the world. People wear shoes to avoid puncture wounds and get tetanus shots to stay a step ahead of the bacteria. Even in Kenya, where more Samburu wear shoes and aid organizations give out tetanus shots, the disease has retreated. Today lockjaw is rare, yet this tradition to remedy it remains.

That afternoon, I thought about that—about how often after a problem no longer needs solving, we still insist on solving it anyway. Or how when a custom is no longer necessary, and can even be harmful or wasteful, we still continue to do it, generation after generation, simply because someone told us to. Bruce liked to tell a story about a woman who always cut the ends off her roast. When asked why, she said it was how her mother did it. Her mother cut the ends off because her mother did it too. When someone asked the grandmother about the practice, she said she cut the ends off because she didn't have a roasting pan big enough. The granddaughter had a new pan that was more than adequate to fit the full roast, but she still threw away food to solve a problem that hadn't applied to her family for two generations.

I wondered how often this happened in other areas—places where we think we're making rational decisions based on current circumstances when instead we're making irrational or inaccurate ones based on old information. How often, for example, do Western doctors and patients alike commit to a "solution" and stick to it long after the problem is solved and treatment is no longer required? For example, Dr. Lee advocated interferons on the basis of an MRI from one year earlier. Maybe a more recent picture would tell a different story.

Was this the case with my mom too? She and I, it seemed, reacted to each other on the basis of actions taken and assumptions we'd made long ago. She was angry because of an old assumption that I'd somehow been able but unwilling to control my health issues when I was younger—that I'd used them to punish or embarrass or hurt her (although I couldn't imagine she really believed I was diagnosed to hurt her). I, in turn, was afraid to talk to her, because I was afraid of repeating a pattern that we'd established in my childhood and perpetuated. I was afraid to disappoint her yet again.

In Africa, for Michelle and me at least, there were no old patterns at play. The heat was so serious it made immediate demands—and that was eye opening and refreshing. During the day, the temperature forced us to sit still for great chunks of time. We stayed by our huts near the bend in the dry riverbed, watching the herders come with their animals each morning and drinking sugary tea with Lepikayo and his friends in the shade of an acacia tree. In the early afternoons, we'd eat a meal, usually rice with boiled carrots and cabbage, the only meal of the day unless Lepikayo decided to kill a goat that he and his friends would cook over the fire. Michelle and I tried to teach them English, and I learned a few phrases in Samburu. *Kay deh deh* means "it is true." *Ashee olaing*, "thank you."

One afternoon, Michelle and I took a walk up the dry riverbed. We saw monkeys in the trees and a family of warthogs on the far bank. The warthogs—which were happily trotting along—saw us and froze in their tracks. We did too. And then, as if on cue, the whole family of beasts lifted their tails and sprinted back into the brush.

Michelle and I walked on. After about a half hour, we came upon a muddy puddle, eight feet across and too murky to see how deep. The brackish water was green and black with some oily substance smeared across the surface.

"One time, I was hiking with Lepikayo and we sat down near a pool like this," Michelle said. "He started taking off his clothes like he was going to dive in so I said, 'Oh no, you can't do that.' I told him all about bacteria that lived in the water, and I explained how the bacteria would get in his mouth, into his intestines and make him sick. I explained as much as I knew about drinking clean water and antibiotics and how to stay healthy."

She continued, "I talked for a while and I thought he was really listening to me, that I was doing a good deed, you know, helping him to stay healthy. And when I was done talking, he looked at me and said, 'That is not my belief system,' and dove in."

"Did he get sick?" I asked.

"No," she said. "And I never brought it up again."

We started walking back to camp, and as we slowly retraced our steps, I thought about how much I loved that story. "That is not my belief system," I repeated. What a handy tool to have in my toolbox.

That night, as I looked at the African sky, I felt small yet strengthened by the endless sea of stars. Each was immense and powerful, shining all alone, and part of a far greater constellation. Looking at such a big picture before me—an endless expanse of sparkling information—it was so easy to see how limited a view I normally had. Even when I can't see all the stars, or know all the answers, I realized, I can trust that they are there and have faith that this universe and all that's in it is really well designed.

## CHAPTER 19

# A REAL DISCONNECT

Sitting in Heathrow, midway between Nairobi and Denver, I texted Bruce to see if he was around. "Hey, sweetie, I'm in London. If you are too, I'll reschedule my next flight and come hang out with you for a few days." He wrote back that he was in Amsterdam on his way to Suriname for some new massive deal he was putting together.

"So you're feeling better?" I wrote. "That's good." No need and no reason to state the obvious: flying to Nairobi was too much, but South America, not a problem.

Bruce texted that he and his doctor had sorted out whatever was making his belly hurt. "It was a value problem," he wrote, and moments later added, "I mean valve problem."

"Value, valve," I replied. "It's all the same. It's about what gets in and what's kept out. Have yourself a ball in Suriname."

After I sent the message, I read it again. "Have yourself a ball in Suriname" sounded like poor cover for "Go fuck yourself in Suriname," and neither was what I actually meant. I wasn't necessarily wishing Bruce a jolly good time there. He would have whatever kind of time he was going to have (I don't know that he ever had a ball doing anything, in fact). But sending him anger felt equally off base because I wasn't angry. Bruce was who he was. And in the end, I was absolutely fine with that. It occurred to me that he liked to swoop in when someone was in crisis and help that person out, try to save people at whatever cost. He'd done that with his ex-wife during her illness, and he'd done that for me through this whole year of fear. When I thought I might be sick and would suffer greatly and alone, Bruce said not a chance: "Whatever it is, we'll take care of it." He stood like a sentinel, saying, "Nothing bad will happen on my watch, and you, Jody, are on my watch." I will be eternally grateful to him for that.

Now, when we were both pretty sure that I was healing (or healed!), he'd moved on to other people, other places, other dramas. He didn't say he was done with me, that he wanted to change or end our relationship. He just would become less available and wander off. I understood where we stood, and for the first time, I accepted it.

*Have yourself a ball in Suriname*, I thought, and I meant it, as I wandered off myself in search of food.

At Heathrow, it wasn't hard. The airport offered all kinds of pleasures I'd missed in Africa. I found a restaurant and inhaled a fresh, green and leafy salad, then I walked to another and savored cold, sweet and creamy ice cream. And finally, I bought the London *Times*, a heavy dose of solid news and analysis, before boarding the next flight.

Eight hours later, I landed in Denver and had to remember where I'd left my car. It seemed so long ago. I found it, picked Riley up from my friend's and pointed my trusty Jeep for home. I unpacked, showered and tried to stay awake until a reasonable hour. I failed and nodded off around seven thirty.

The next morning, wide awake at four in the morning, I made

myself wait several hours to call Lisa to let her know I was home safe. I went to the post office to pick up my mail, and leafing through the pile of magazines and junk, I found a small envelope from Dr. Lee. I opened it and read that it was "a pleasure" to see me in the office. Her experience was different from mine, clearly.

"There is a real disconnect between the clinical symptoms and the findings on the MRI," she wrote and briefly recapped what I had told her about the now nonexistent tingling. "The only other symptoms are a slight sensation of decreased strength in the left foot that only identified today in testing when you first went on to the ball of the right foot and then onto the left."

*Why not say I can balance longer on my right foot?* I kept reading.

"Your history is notable for an absence of many symptoms, including weakness or further sensory symptoms in the upper and lower extremities as well as an absence of visual symptoms," she wrote.

*Call me crazy, but doesn't an absence of symptoms point to an absence of disease? What do I know? I'm no neurologist.*

The MRI, Dr. Lee wrote, "favored a diagnosis of multiple sclerosis" and led to her list of recommendations, which included getting a microbial evaluation of my gut, calling her Buddhist teacher for support and making an appointment with the MS specialists at the university.

She signed her name in a large scrawl and below that, she noted that she had CC'ed Dr. Maureen Duncan.

*Ridiculous*, I thought. I had filled out the HIPAA release form and wrote very clearly to send results only to me. In person, I had told her twice more to send the results to me and no one else. Still, she copied Dr. Duncan.

She didn't listen to me, and as I reread the letter and reconsidered what she was telling me, I realized she didn't listen to herself either. She had conducted a two-hour interview and an extensive physical exam and dismissed the results because they did not confirm the image of a $3,000 snapshot taken one year ago. Her three-dimensional, full-color, surround-sound, live experience was less important than the silent black-and-white picture on a computer screen. Her time and what she saw, heard and felt meant less than a test ordered by another neurologist who she thought "hadn't done his work emotionally."

It was as if she were focusing very closely on just one star and excluding all the others in the galaxy.

I went to my filing cabinet, dropped her letter in my medical folder and kicked the drawer shut. Never believed in the tooth fairy anyway.

I wondered if I believed in doctors at all. I thought about my earliest memories and all those years as a kid when my mom said, "Fix her," as she handed me to one doctor or another, as if the doctors were powerful and perfect and I was neither. I thought about all the times I struggled to trust my experience—with the shrink and the stomachaches, with the orthodontists and ultimately with Dr. Silver—all the times I wondered whether they might be right and I didn't really feel what I thought I felt.

Was I doing it still? I'd just spent a year touring the American medical landscape—and hating nearly every minute of it—and I had two more doctors' appointments in my calendar, both booked before I went to Africa. I had a follow-up with Dr. Desai and an appointment with an osteopath a friend recommended because osteopaths are systems thinkers. They look at a bigger picture and see how pieces interrelate. Still, I contemplated canceling her and Desai. Then, I contemplated keeping both, considering what I hoped to get out of either. And while I didn't know, I was curious.

In the end, I kept the osteopath almost by default: I never made the call to cancel.

On a sunny morning in mid-February, I followed the directions to a quiet street in Boulder. I walked the stairs to her second-story office and took a seat on a wicker chair in the small waiting area. She had old magazines in a basket and books on gardening. Soon, I heard movement behind the closed door. When the door opened, a shortish barefoot woman said good-bye to a taller blond.

"Jody?" the barefoot woman asked. "I'm Jillian, go on in."

I went in and as soon as Jillian joined me, I exploded into a speed talker's version of my year of fear, rattling on and on about doctors and terror and tests. I fired away as if I had to get out all the words before I ran out of air. Midway through my torrent of words, Jillian said, "All right, stand up. Let's have a look."

Blond and wearing dark-framed glasses, Jillian was curvy and looked very Boulder—comfy clothing and no makeup. She turned me around, put her hands on my shoulders and felt along my spine. "Lay down," she said, motioning to the massage table. "On your back."

I looked at the ceiling, and she took a seat at the head of the table. She ran her hands under my shoulders and moved them around as my mouth continued firing at full speed. "What do you think lesions mean? Do you think they're still there? Do you think they've gone away? Do you think they mean anything at all? What's osteopathy? And what's craniosacral osteopathy?"

Jillian continued to work on my back, and as best she could, she tried to answer my barrage of questions until suddenly, there was no need. I might have been midquestion when I abruptly fell into a deep, deep sleep. Just like that, lights out. Jillian continued to do her thing. And maybe twenty minutes later, I was nudged out of sleep by a loud buzzing sound, rhythmic and far away. In my slumber, I thought I was in a large, cavernous room like an empty gymnasium, and I wondered where. I wondered who was snoring on the other side, maybe twenty or thirty feet from me, who had nodded out under the bleachers. I kept my eyes shut and tried to figure out where I was when I realized the sound was coming from my own nostrils.

They seemed so far away. Or else I had been.

Feeling slightly confused and mostly embarrassed, I opened my eyes and saw that Jillian had slid over the side of the table and had her hands under my lumbar spine.

"Wow," I said. "I musta fallen asleep."

She smiled.

After a while, she said, "OK, Jody. Take your time getting up."

I drove home feeling different. I had no idea what just happened, not intellectually anyway. But physically, my body understood that something dramatic had shifted. Places in my body that I hadn't known were tight—like my jaw—suddenly felt softer, less rigid. And my upper back, that spot behind my heart and between my shoulder blades, felt bigger, more expansive, like there was more room and more mobility.

At home, I walked Riley, worked through the afternoon, made dinner, tried to read and went to bed early, falling asleep without time to think about it. Just out. In the morning, everything still felt different and warm like later afternoon when the sun bathed everything in warmth. And it was only seven—hours and hours before the golden hour.

I knew I would see Jillian again. The decision wasn't even a decision, not a conscious, rational conclusion. I knew I'd go see her again like I knew I'd eat lunch. I knew in my bones and in my cells that whatever she did was beneficial, necessary even. And that she was

"I know. I'm not that fun to eat with on this diet."

"It's only a week, right?"

"Three."

"Oh shit. Good luck with that."

Thankfully, she came over anyway.

When the three weeks were over, I boiled an egg, ate it and continued on the no-nothing diet for a couple days to see if I reacted to the egg. Nothing happened so I tried dairy and waited for three days. No reaction there either, so I moved on to gluten. For dinner, I boiled pasta and tossed it with olive oil, lemon and parsley. All in all, the meal was boring and bland but the texture felt familiar and soothing and almost foreign after four weeks without it.

The next morning, before I even got out of bed I knew something was wrong. My body ached like I'd been in a car wreck that I couldn't recall. I hadn't. I took Riley for a walk and didn't feel any better. I came home, fed the pup, stretched a little and sat down to meditate. Sitting cross-legged on the floor felt like hell. I could hardly focus on my breathing because my hips were screaming. Same for my ankles and feet. When I stood up, I realized there were other problems. My knees were sore, my shoulders felt wrong, my low back was tight and even my elbows were squawking like something had happened to them.

I showered and went out into the world, thinking a change of venue would help. I had a consulting project and decided to work at the Tattered Cover. Bookstores are like Disneyland for me—the happiest place on earth. With all those books and thoughts and carefully chosen words, there's no room for bad feelings or ugly actions. Or at least that's what I thought until I walked in. The guy at the counter said hello and I scowled at him.

It was like flipping off Mickey Mouse but I couldn't help myself.

I went to the coffee counter, ordered a cup of mint tea and found a table in the front room. At another table, two women were talking about a television show. I nearly turned to glare at them like they were invading my private office. *Yikes, what am I doing?*

I got through the day without picking a fight, though several times I felt the urge. I crawled in bed early because all my joints still ached and lying down seemed like the only good option. I slept fitfully and woke the next day still uncomfortable—a little less achy but still achy. I didn't add any more new foods that day or the next. After a few days, when I felt normal again, I went to a diner for lunch and ordered scrambled eggs, no toast, no home fries—just a side of fruit and cup of decaf.

By the time I stood up, I felt like I'd downed a Red Bull or twenty. I couldn't sit still, couldn't focus, couldn't stay with any thought or conversation.

I went home and tried to unwind. When my brain settled, I got some work done. And in the evening, when I was ready to eat again, I cooked rice and sautéed vegetables in olive oil. I ate nothing more interesting than that for the next four days until I could see Dr. Desai.

Inside her office, sitting next to her in the big comfy chair, I told her that gluten felt like a car wreck and that caffeine, or the little bit of it in the decaf, made me want to jump out of my skin.

"Good to know," she said. "You should stay off gluten and avoid caffeine." Her smile was the same sweet and inclusive grin. *We're both seeing the logic here, right?* And yeah, we were, almost.

"A gluten intolerance or sensitivity could explain a lot of things—the reason you felt bloated after meals your whole life, the intestinal distress throughout your childhood, the chronic constipation you've experienced," Dr. Desai said.

"It could also cause malabsorption, which would explain the

vitamin deficiencies, even the tingling in the fingertips and toes," she added. She then checked my pulse in one wrist and said, "Oh yeah, you're colon is much happier now."

"Wait," I said. "How could gluten be the answer? I've been tested for celiac disease. I'm sure of it. And the test came back negative."

"A blood test?" she asked. I nodded and she continued, "There are false positives and false negatives. And, really, what do you think is a better diagnostic tool? A lab test or your own body?"

And finally, *finally*, her logic won me over. "When you put it that way…It's funny, you know, I was so mad that Dr. Lee deferred to the MRI, like it was a better test than my body. Now that I think about it, that wasn't the first time. I was annoyed that Silver thought the test was more important than me explaining how I actually felt—especially when the drugs worsened my symptoms and then I got better after stopping them. Same for Duncan with the heavy metal test and the chelation that made me feel so lousy. And yet, I did the chelation for months, trusting the test results more than what my body was telling me…Faith in technology and medical testing—those are tough habits to break!"

We sat for a moment until another thought popped into my head.

"So how does this work?" I asked. "How does gluten gum up everything?"

Dr. Desai explained that for people who can't tolerate gluten, consuming it irritates the lining of their intestines. And when the lining is irritated, the intestine can't function properly. In some people, the body reacts to gluten by trying to release the contents of the colon quickly—my life as a kid summed up right there!—and in others, the body holds on to food too long, or my life as an adult. And over time, if the person keeps eating gluten, it irritates the very fine gaps in the intestine where broken-down food enters the bloodstream. The very fine gaps grow larger, making poorer gatekeepers. Larger particles slip through the gaps and travel with the blood throughout the body. Because the body recognizes the undigested particles as foreign objects, the body creates an immune response that then attacks the undigested gluten. In other words, the body looks like it's starting to attack itself.

Bingo! "Oh," I said, "I can't believe that all of my issues stem from a teeny, tiny valve problem. What gets in and what stays out. I think that's what Dr. Lee was talking about when she said I had leaky gut."

"Yes," Dr. Desai said. "And when the intestine's not working properly, it's difficult for the body to absorb the nutrients it needs from foods."

That would also explain all the weird nutrient deficiency results I'd had. I was flabbergasted. "I can't believe that basically everything that has been plaguing me over the years since my childhood, and especially this year, is ultimately due to a serious gluten problem."

Dr. Desai took the pulses in my other wrist, reading the signs from an Ayurvedic perspective. "Hmm," she said. "Your *vata*'s still pushing *pitta*."

Dr. Desai wanted to balance my *doshas*—we both did—so she outlined her plan to get me there. It included vitamins B and D, fish oil and the herb *ashwangandha*. We talked about *abhyanga*, of self-massage, and I said I would try that too. She also suggested I make fennel tea to settle my stomach and take a probiotic at night. Sure thing, I said, and agreed to do it all and return in two months.

Over the next few weeks, I returned to the bookstore (kinder and calmer now—no more scowling at the nice man at the desk) to learn more about my gut. I found *Celiac Disease: a Hidden Epidemic*, by Dr. Peter H. R. Green and Rory Jones. I didn't even have to open the book to see that tingling in the extremities is a common symptom of gluten issues. The good doctors listed common signs on the back cover. *Wonder why neurologists don't start there?* I wondered. *Why pull out the big guns like an expensive and terrifying MRI? Why deliver the nasty and forever diagnosis when gluten could be the culprit?*

Fired up, I kept digging. In *The Inside Tract: Your Good Gut Guide to Great Digestive Health*, by Dr. Gerard E. Mullin and Kathie Madonna Swift (MS, RD, LDN), I read how involuntary muscle twitches sent Mullin to neurologists who gave him terrifying answers. The MS specialist said MS and suggested a lumbar puncture to test Mullen's spinal fluid. The test sent him into searing pain. The fix for the pain, a blood patch, gave him a painful disease called arachnoiditis. The "cure" for the arachnoiditis, intravenous steroids, left him with cardiac arrhythmia, ulcers and an immune system so suppressed that it opened the door for pneumonia. He didn't have MS but in search of it, he suffered all kinds of other doctor-induced trauma. This downward spiral left Mullins, a world-renowned gastroenterologist, at "the end of the road with Western medicine."

And this was a guy who had traveled that road long enough to graduate from medical school, complete an internship and residency, open a practice, and see patients for a dozen years. I'd only taken a few steps and found the path crowded with fear and panic and reasons to pull off.

I also found that I wasn't alone. In addition to Mullin, everyone I knew, it seemed, knew someone who had been misdiagnosed with MS. Real culprits included misdiagnosed Lyme disease, a benign tumor on the spinal cord, the lingering effects of a car wreck and—yep—gluten sensitivity.

In *Overdiagnosed: Making People Sick in the Pursuit of Health*, Dr. H. Gilbert Welch wrote about a clinic where many patients suffered sinus pain. Doctors routinely ordered X-rays of the facial sinuses, and nearly every film came back with a diagnosis of sinusitis. To check the veracity of this decree, Dr. Welch ordered an X-ray of his own face, and despite having no symptoms, he was diagnosed with sinusitis.

"Our diagnostic technologies are of such high resolution that we are discovering more ambiguities and more surprise abnormalities," he wrote, adding that the ambiguities and abnormalities lead to more testing, more scanning, more ambiguities and more treatment—even as the patient remains asymptomatic.

"While relatively few people are said to have disease when doctors examine their outsides," Welch wrote, "relatively many are said to have disease when scanners examine their insides."

Welch concluded that overdiagnosis leads "millions of people to become patients unnecessarily, to be treated needlessly, and to bear the inconvenience and financial burdens associated with overdiagnosis."

I understood. And felt like I had dodged a bullet. Because Dr. Silver didn't address my questions or ever return my calls, I went into stubborn reporter mode and found answers. And out of habit, I kept searching. And I kept finding reasons to rule out the MRI.

In my favorite study, a widely known sports medicine doctor sent thirty-one healthy professional athletes—baseball pitchers with no pain and superhuman throwing arms—to get MRIs. These men hurled a ball upward of ninety miles an hour and almost all of their scans said to operate. The test showed abnormalities in 90 percent of the "patients."

In *Selling Sickness: How the World's Biggest Pharmaceutical Companies Are Turning Us All into Patients*, Ray Moynihan and Alan Cassels explain one possible reason for the abundance of medical diagnoses. In gruesome detail, they report ways drug companies manipulate data and doctors to fulfill the companies' fiduciary duties to shareholders.

As I read, I reconsidered my thoughts about the two neurologists who were so committed to the same MRI and MS drugs. In my mind, and in conversations with friends, I had cursed them both and called them stupid and mean and lazy, but I've come to realize that, like most doctors, they're probably smart, well-intentioned people who entered medical school because they wanted to help people. Throughout their coursework, residencies, internships and other training, they learned of valuable tools including the latest and greatest technologies, intricate pharmaceutical therapies and surgical interventions. And like many doctors, they probably received little to no education on food and nutrition and how those two factors can affect a person's health in other areas. If the law of the instrument says "To a man with a hammer, every problem looks like a nail," then the opposite must be true too. If food and nutrition aren't in the toolbox, they can't be the solution.

Time is also an issue. Dietary solutions are rarely immediately visible and take time to diagnose—time that physicians don't always have with their patients. Nationally, primary care doctors see an average of twenty-five patients a day. If they worked ten hours and spent all their time with those patients—no lunch, no paperwork, no bathroom break—they'd have twenty-four minutes with each patient. That's all, just twenty-four minutes to listen, explain, evaluate, answer questions and make recommendations. And while they're already crunched for time, there's also a slew of outside pressures pushing them toward the seemingly quicker solution of prescribing pills: persuasive salespeople, forceful marketing campaigns and favorable data on drugs, all of which pharmaceutical companies frequently sponsor or manipulate. That can be a lot to stand up against.

Furthermore, doctors are told they are special—superior even—just by virtue of getting into medical school. This can lend itself to a serious sense of superiority and overconfidence in their own opinions, ideas and solutions. Then, they spend years and years learning the latest, greatest gadgets and keeping up with the newest chemical compounds. They are trained to diagnose, and when they complete their schooling, they are licensed and paid to do the same. Well-respected, well-known neurologists are pretty much loaded for bear. With all their accumulated knowledge and technology, swatting a fly can't be that fun. And gluten, smaller than a fly, is something the patient can handle on her own—no doctor needed. No billing code to jot down.

Still dangerously and endlessly curious, I pulled out the one-pagers Silver gave me. I called each pharmaceutical company and asked for more information. I said I had been diagnosed with MS, which was true, and that I was considering taking their drug, which was not. I said I'd like to know more about each drug and wondered if they could send me the original study that was referenced on the pages I held. Each company's representative said there was no more information, not for me. One said, "If you have your doctor call with the request, we might be able to send him the study."

"Him?" I asked, incredulously, as if the sexist assumption were the only crime.

These companies were selling something to alter brain chemistry, and they acted as if a potential buyer would just say, "Oh, OK," and swallow the pill—or inject the prescription, in this case—without asking any questions. That's not how my brain works. I assumed if they didn't want to show their hand, they had something to hide.

And that excited me. I was a journalist once. I had investigative skills. I wanted to flex them. And honestly, it didn't seem that hard. Drug studies done for FDA approval are public information.

From the comfort of my own desk, I went to the National

Institutes of Health PubMed database and searched "Betaseron," one of the drugs recommended. Among the first citations was this from the *British Medical Journal*: "Why Interferon Beta 1b Was Licensed Is a Mystery." The author wrote that the drug "has been shown to reduce the rate of relapse in relapsing multiple sclerosis by one third and to diminish the accretion of disease as shown by magnetic resonance imaging. Unfortunately, neither of these two variables has any convincing relation to disability."

The scans, in the author's experience, showed no relationship to disability. He mentioned patients "who seem on magnetic resonance imaging to have no brains left, who lead full and active lives"—asymptomatic lesions in other words—and patients with severe disability "whose scans apparently show trivial disease."

I spent four or five hours searching the database and found nothing that seemed a compelling argument for the drugs.

I felt vindicated, a little restless and eager to spread the news. How many people are like me? How many people are quickly diagnosed based on an MRI that doesn't correlate to the physical reality? Silver said MS was the most common diagnosis he gave to women. How many doctors are like him? And how many diagnoses are really misdiagnoses?

I called the Rocky Mountain MS Society and said I was a journalist writing about my diagnosis. I asked if there was someone I could speak to, and the receptionist suggested Pat Daly, the director of counseling and support services.

We scheduled a meeting, and I prepped like I was prepping for an interview with an NFL coach. I scoured newspaper stories, magazine articles and books; I made phone calls; I searched the MS Society's website; and I reread notes taken throughout my adventures in Healthcareland. I wrote questions, read them and wrote more. I scavenged libraries and bookstores, and found Ann Boroch's *Healing Multiple Sclerosis* and Elaine DeLack's *They Say It Didn't Make Cents: MS and the Prokarin Story*.

Both women experienced serious symptoms that were diagnosed as MS and both cured themselves in different ways. And while I was thrilled with these two, I found an even more appealing woman on YouTube: Dr. Terry Wahls, who gave a TED Talk called "Minding My Mitochondria."

An internal medicine physician, Wahls was diagnosed with MS in 2000. She had access to the best doctors and the latest and greatest medicine available. She tried chemotherapy and other immune-suppressant drugs and still slid from walking to a wheel chair in four years. Frustrated, Wahls conducted her own research and radically changed her diet—avoiding most grains—to alter her mitochondria, which she called "the power plants that keep our cells going."

"Aren't they beautiful?" she said as she marched, energetically and unassisted, around the stage, waving her arms and pointing to a picture of translucent blobby oval. As Wahls talked she also showed photos of herself—first in a judo pose, then in a zero-gravity wheelchair, where she couldn't lift her head, and finally, after overhauling her diet, riding a bike and sitting, smiling, on a horse.

I made a mental note to call Christopher, my skinny guide back in Vancouver. He had suggested I find people who did what I wanted to do and follow them. These women were it, having blazed a trail. They knew that nothing was forever—not sickness, not sadness, not even belief systems. Wahls was a great example. She believed in diagnoses and doctors. And she lay down, took all that Western medicine could offer, tossed her assumptions aside, devised her own plan and got back up. She was proof that the human body could move in many directions—toward ease, away from disease, sideways, upward and onward.

A body can fall out of balance and find it again.

# CHAPTER 20

# EXPERTS SAY

The sky was wide, open and blue as I drove to the Rocky Mountain MS Society for my interview. And my optimism was nearly as big.

This interview, I believed, was going to cap this year of searching. The MS Society would know about MRIs, misdiagnoses, Terry Wahls—a doctor who had healed and explained how in a TED Talk—and how diet affects health and well-being. They would know that gluten sensitivities can mimic symptoms of MS and that one MRI without clinical findings was more of a Rorschach test than anything definitive or damning.

The MS Society, and its Colorado branch, I assumed, would be staffed by experts in all things related to MS. In my mind at least, they would be on the cutting edge of understanding, or at least compiling the various stories of people like me.

I pulled into the parking lot of an old school, and before I got out of the car, I watched a woman trying to load men and women in wheelchairs into a short bus as if they were cattle. I felt for them and felt the pull again of that small sliver of fear that maybe I had it too. That maybe the MRI was right and everything I learned was wrong. I wondered if, after all of the crazy things I'd done over this year, this was my dumbest idea ever.

I went in anyway. Time to settle this matter once and for all.

Inside the building in Westminster, a peaceful suburb where people walk their dogs on wide paths and city council members post their home phone numbers online, the receptionist sat behind bulletproof glass. She buzzed the door so I could walk around and talk to her face-to-face, over a counter without the glass. She was sitting at a long desk at the end of a long room. Behind her, in the big, open space that may have been the school lunchroom at one time, twenty or thirty people whirled around in motorized wheel chairs. I told the receptionist I had an appointment to interview the society's spokesperson, Pat Daly. The receptionist pointed me to a bank of offices off the hall.

I walked the length of the building and took a seat to wait. After a few minutes, Pat asked me into her office. It was small with a big desk and two chairs facing each other.

For a moment, I wondered what I was I thinking when I made this appointment. Then I looked down at the notebook in my lap. *Oh, right—I'm a reporter.* Other people in situations like mine may not have the skills or stubbornness that it took for me to find the right diagnosis, the right treatment, and the right doctor or expert who could help. Throughout my journey, I'd come to realize how many people get locked into misdiagnoses and then have to suffer the consequences. After everything that I had been through, I had taken charge of my own health, and I was determined to help others who have been misdiagnosed, undiagnosed, underdiagnosed or even overdiagnosed become their own self-advocates for their health. I would ask questions for them. And I'd start with an easy one: "How did you get started working here?"

Pat told me she'd been working for the society for years and had left for a while but came back.

"Is it challenging working with MS patients when it's such a scary disease and so difficult to diagnose?"

"No, it's not," she said and looked at me like I was not very bright. "It's not difficult to diagnose."

Wondering what I was missing, I said, "What do you mean?"

"I've been here for years and I've never, not once, heard of anyone being de-diagnosed."

"You never heard of anyone who was diagnosed with MS and then found out it was something else?" I asked.

"No, never," she said.

*Interesting*, I thought.

But, Daly added, life had become much better for those diagnosed since the disease-modifying drugs came into existence. She asked if I was on them and when I said no, she suggested I start on them quickly. Research, she said, shows that people have better results if they start taking the drugs straight away.

"I hadn't heard that," I said. "Do you have that research?"

"No but it's a public document. I'm sure you can find it."

*That's helpful.*

As I began to discuss the Mayo Clinic's website, which said that many patients do really well without taking drugs, she barely let me finish. "That must be old information," she said.

"So the patients did well, but in retrospect you think they didn't?" I asked.

"Look," she said, "you don't understand MS. I've got a cartoon on my computer that will help."

She spun the computer screen so we both could see it and opened a file with a red and green drawing of the brain. There was a yellow spot on the surface that represented a lesion.

"See, as MS progresses, the lesion eats up brain cells—*click, click,*

*click, click, click*—like Pac-Man," she said, cheerfully imitating the noise of the video game.

"*Click, click, click*," she continued, using her hand like a snapping bird to demonstrate how the MS (Pac-Man) would eat brain tissue. She clicked to the next picture, which showed the same red and green brain with a much bigger yellow spot. And on the third picture, the lesion had grown even bigger and the brain had grown smaller inside the cartoon skull.

"Over time, the brain gets smaller and smaller and smaller," she said, a bit too cheerfully.

I inhaled deeply and looked down at the note pad in my lap.

"Yes, the brain shrinks, eventually to the size of a raisin. And that leads to greater disability."

I don't know how I got through the rest of the interview. What a dark world she described, where everything moves inescapably toward chaos and pain. And at this point, I already knew that wasn't my world. I also knew what she was saying wasn't true for me.

After all, I had been searching for a year for my own answers. I heard different theories and different belief systems and had finally arrived at the truth: there isn't one right answer that is true and right for everyone.

One ugly MRI did not mean take the drugs and accept the disease. It didn't mean that for me—or for Ann Boroch or Elaine DeLack or Terry Wahls, the women who'd been diagnosed and had devised their own cures. If an MRI and MS diagnosis weren't the end of the story for us, then they didn't have to mean the same thing for everyone.

And yet the woman who spoke to MS patients for the Rocky Mountain MS Society seemed to argue that an MRI was infallible; that lesions undeniably mean MS; and that in the case of an ugly MRI, there were only two choices: drugs or declining health.

Feeling like I'd heard enough, I wrapped up the interview quickly. And as I drove away, I wondered how many "experts" were locked into the same narrow logic and how many patients had been harmed by that.

I continued researching the disease and eventually found three MS specialists—board-certified, highly respected neurologists—at the Oregon Health and Science University who were seeing so many misdiagnoses in their practices that they became curious. They wondered, much like I did, how many patients are saddled with a label that doesn't fit. They sent a survey to their peers across the country and asked if others also saw a lot of misdiagnoses. Nearly everyone, 97 percent, had seen at least one patient in the previous year with a long-standing misdiagnosis. A majority had seen more than five. Two-thirds of the doctors surveyed said informing a patient of their misdiagnosis was challenging, and about one in seven, or 14 percent, said they chose not to tell the patient at all.

The last part was staggering: 14 percent of MS specialists saw a patient who believed he or she had MS, determined that it wasn't MS and chose not to tell the patient.

Astonished, I called one of the authors asking for an explanation. "MS is a clinical diagnosis," said Dr. Dennis Bourdette. "It requires a lot of experience and people don't take the time."

On the survey, the doctors could select from several reasons for not informing the patient. Some feared the truth could cause psychological harm or a loss of support. But in choosing not to inform the patient, the doctors would never know if the news would cause psychological harm. And even if they worried that the patient would no longer be eligible for disability payments, payments are made on the basis of disability, not the label. If there were reasons other than MS that a patient couldn't work, the patient still wouldn't be able to work and would still be eligible for financial support. So that couldn't be a reason for them not to inform their patients.

Other doctors surveyed felt the referring physician should break the news, or that the news didn't need to be broken because the diagnosis was benign.

*Benign*? I was nearly breathless when I read that. *Benign*? If patients are experiencing symptoms of some sort and are being treated for something they don't have, then they're *not* being treated for something they *do* have. In my case, for example, I was told I had MS when in fact the issue was a gluten intolerance. If one of the other doctors I saw had determined this later but chosen not to tell me, I would have continued eating gluten indefinitely, causing more damage to my intestines and making me feel worse and worse, with no end in sight. And if I had taken the interferon drugs, which research shows only work in about one-third of the patients, I might have resigned myself to declining health and said, "Well, I tried."

I called Dr. Andrew Solomon, who coauthored the study. He was as generous with his time as Bourdette was, and just as understanding about how angry this study made me.

"One in seven?" I asked.

"I'm an MS specialist," Solomon said. "So I see MS and not MS all day long. Other neurologists, where it's a small part of their practice, don't have the same experience.

"I think people overinterpret the MRI," he said. "And there's an overreliance on the test."

He told me that he, Bourdette and the third author—Dr. Eran Klein—were committed to more research. More studies could be published in more journals and presented at more conferences to reach more neurologists. And if more neurologists understood the intricacies of diagnosing MS, that may lessen the risk of overdiagnosis and lead to better patient care overall.

"I'm grateful you're looking into it," I told Dr. Solomon. "I really am."

I was and remain grateful that these three doctors are thought leaders in the world of MS and that they are on the case to uncover misdiagnoses and improve patient outcomes. And I wish their reach were bigger than the MS world. Research shows that as many as one in five of all diagnoses, across all categories, are misdiagnoses. One report found that the number of fatal diagnostic errors in intensive-care units in the United States equals the number of deaths related to breast cancer each year—40,500.

In his bestselling book *How Doctors Think*, Dr. Jerome Groopman calls misdiagnosis "a window into the medical mind." He reviewed recent studies that show medical errors are caused more often by flawed thinking than technical mistakes.

"In one study of misdiagnoses that caused serious harm to patients," Groopman writes, "some 80 percent could be accounted for by a cascade of cognitive errors, like the one in [a specific patient's] case, putting her into a narrow frame and ignoring information that contradicted a fixed notion."

Unfortunately, the problem affects all of us. As a group, Americans spend nearly $2.8 trillion on health care each year. By some estimates, preventable medical error is the sixth-leading cause of death in the United States. The enormity of the problem made me shudder. What is the cost of unnecessary treatment, overtreatment and error because we (or our doctors) are racing to find a quick fix?

✚ ✚ ✚

"What have you done to yourself?"

Jillian, the craniosacral osteopath, stood behind me as I looked out the windows in her office. She hadn't touched my back yet and was only eyeballing me.

"You're tight and twisted in your lower back. There's tension in your neck and between your shoulders. What did you do?"

"Um, nothing," I said. "Nothing I can think of."

I lay down on the table, and Jillian slid her hands under my shoulders. She asked me what I'd been up to, and I said I'd started writing about my adventures, or misadventures, in Healthcareland. "I'm a writer," I said, "and writing is how I've always made sense of the world. And the whole world of medicine, diagnoses and doctors was so bewildering, it was like a foreign planet, orbiting some other sun."

Jillian listened as she pressed on points between ribs and along my spine, gently and efficiently unleashing the tension she found.

"I feel like I crash-landed on this crazy planet and needed to write to find my way home."

"That's good for you," Jillian said, continuing to find and relieve spots that I hadn't even realized were tender.

Writing now made sense. I had been reporting—almost unknowingly—for a year since the debacle with Dr. Silver. I had started asking questions because it's what I do and because I was scared. Instinctually, I'd started gathering bits of information like so many bricks that I could use to build a barricade between me and his gloomy diagnosis. As I went from doctor to doctor and flew to Canada, California and back to Denver, I had collected information and ideas about interconnections of body, mind and spirit. Or more accurately, I had learned how *my* body, mind and spirit were connected. More than connected, they were in fact the same thing. All one. And I finally started writing as a way of making sense of this understanding and sharing what I had learned.

"As part of my research, I went to the Rocky Mountain MS Society last week," I told Jillian. "It was awful. The receptionist sat behind bulletproof glass—like they thought they were going to be attacked and needed to keep scary people out, or maybe sick people in—and the social worker told me she'd never heard of anyone being de-diagnosed, though I've found serious evidence to the contrary. And she showed me drawings of brains and said mine would shrink to the size of a—"

"Jody," Jillian cut me off. "What were you thinking? You cannot do things like that. When I asked what did you do to yourself, this is the answer. Going there is what you did to yourself."

She was right and I knew it. I just didn't want to believe that I could fold that easily, that I wasn't invincible, that I was no longer someone who could march unafraid and unaffected into hostile territories like locker rooms filled with NFL giants and small offices manned by medical professionals. Maybe I never could march in and get out unscathed and I just didn't know it.

Jillian's voice moved like her hands—direct, to the point and designed to interrupt bad habits. I looked up to her face and saw she was smiling and shaking her head, the way someone would when training a puppy. The puppy's sweet and lovable and even cute while eating jelly beans, and yet the whole scenario won't lead to anything good.

"It seemed like a good idea at the time," I started and then stopped. I knew she was right and I knew at the time that I shouldn't have gone.

She spent the next forty minutes unleashing the stress that enveloped my spine.

A few weeks later, I saw Dr. Desai, and no surprise, she concurred with Jillian: I should avoid people and places committed to believing in my demise. I knew it too—it's a little like avoiding foods that make me feel sick.

It seemed obvious, and yet there was a time—not too long ago—when it wasn't. I'd spent decades listening to others tell me how to take care of myself. I'd simultaneously mistrusted experts and followed their directions anyway, seriously suffering when they were wrong. As the debate over health care and our health as a nation continues to rage, the pressure to do as we're told, especially in matters of health, continues to increase, and all the machinery—the white coats and diplomas, the absurdly short doctors' appointments, and the implied urgency of drug studies that say, "Take this now or else"—works to ensure that we as patients acquiesce without considering the implications or alternatives that could be healthier for us.

I'd learned to take care of myself because I had my team, my two doctors—an osteopath and an Ayurvedic physician—who were trained to help me work with and listen to my body. I decided to help others find their own best care and to ensure that they and their needs are being supported—and I started by sharing my story here.

## CHAPTER 21

# THE BAY OF BENGAL

In October, I dialed Mitra in Santa Cruz, California, and told her I wanted to join her in India the next time she went. I was ready. I was no longer afraid for my health and still wanted to experience the trip I missed.

I'd been off gluten for nine months and had completed the Ayurvedic herbal remedies that Dr. Desai prescribed. My gut had finally healed from a lifetime of giving it what it didn't want and couldn't use. As a result, my intestinal tract was working and nutrients could make their way from my food, through my gut, into my bloodstream and to every cell in my body, giving them the tools they needed to repair. The tingling was long gone, same for the tightness in my feet. As an added bonus, sensations I never thought of as symptoms disappeared too. Teeny little bumps I'd always had on the back of my arms went away, and during the day my energy level stayed consistently high from the time I awoke to the time I went to bed. I no longer soared and crashed a couple times a day.

And Jillian played a part too. After my first few sessions with her, I fell into a rhythm of seeing her for craniosacral therapy every two weeks for several months and then once a month. And each time, as I lay on that table with her hands under my back, I could feel her encouraging and teaching my body to give up the tension I'd been carrying as long as I could remember. She taught me to physically give up old habits that outlived the problem they were created to solve. I don't know that I'll ever understand the details of how craniosacral osteopathy works, but in many ways it doesn't matter. I don't need to know intellectually because physically, it makes perfect sense.

I told Mitra about Dr. Desai and how she helped me to clean up my diet and eat foods that are nourishing for me, and how Jillian taught me to feel better and calmer in my body.

And finally, I told Mitra I wanted to practice yoga with her in India and to learn about the woman everyone called Mother. Mitra was thrilled and said, yes, we could do that.

✚ ✚ ✚

In January, two years to the date after I started the journey, I boarded the flights I had canceled so long ago. I left Denver, flew through Frankfurt, and landed in Chennai in the middle of a hot and heavy night. I found my luggage and walked outside to learn that, even at one in the morning, people were screaming, car horns were honking and men were frantically waving signs with people's names. I found a sign that said "JODEE, Quiet Healing," and introduced myself.

"I am Shiva," the man said, "I will take you to Auroville."

We drove out of the airport and onto a two-lane road, lit only by the full moon. He told me that my name—he pronounced it with a *T* for the *D*—meant "light" in Hindi. After about an hour, he pulled off the road and parked beneath a bridge. "I'd like to get some chai," he said. "Would you like some?"

I said no, I'd wait in the car. I rolled down the windows and lay down across the backseat, propping my head on my backpack to look through the opposite window at the moon. In no time, a cow stuck her nose in the same window to take a look at me. "What big eyes you have, my dear," I said. And they were huge, dark and wet, like a baby's.

The cow stayed a moment, pulled her head out of the window and ambled away. Shiva returned and drove the rest of the way to the Quiet Healing Center. The place was completely dark and silent. The electricity was still out from a recent storm, so the night watchman gave me a candle and showed me to my room.

In the morning, around six, I awoke and walked outside to see where I was. I followed the gravel path through the gardens and toward the sound of the ocean. I stood watching and listening to the Bay of Bengal crawl up upon the sand and scurry back. I turned and continued on the gravel path, just a few steps, and saw Mitra ahead in one of her flowing, goddesslike dresses. Her hair was pulled into a bun, and her glasses sat perched on top of her head. When I caught up to her, she hugged me wordlessly and tight.

For fourteen of the next nineteen days, I practiced yoga twice a day, two hours at a stretch, alongside men and women from Switzerland, France, Italy, Germany and India. As we held our poses—some of us with ease and grace, others with effort—we listened to Mitra explain the teachings of Sri Aurobindo and the woman who breathed life into his philosophy and built a permanent home for it in Auroville, the woman everyone called Mother.

And she was everywhere. Portraits of the Mother graced a wall in nearly every public space in Auroville. Her sweet, expressive eyes watched over every person who walked through. And her almost smile inspired in me the same feeling I felt with Jillian, Dr. Desai and Mitra. A mother's love, unconditional and pure, is a kind of faith.

In between yoga classes and on days off, I went with Mitra and other students to explore Auroville and Pondicherry, the closest town. One afternoon, I met an elephant named Lakshmi outside a temple to Ganesha, and she blessed me with her trunk. Another day, I went to a street party for Pongol, where men and women threw bananas in the air and chanted, "Pongol, Pongol, Pongol," as cows paraded by with balloons tied to their horns. And one of the final days, I traveled by car to Tiruvannamalai, a fabulous ancient city, where an enormous temple honors Lord Shiva and an ashram provides home to Brahmana and the remains of Ramana Maharshi. I met dozens of backpackers, tourists and travelers who were all in India to spend time with spiritual leaders. Like me, they were on a path to find peace in their bodies and souls.

Every day, and many times a day, I talked to strangers who started sentences with "My guru says..." Each time I asked the name of the guru, I heard a different answer.

India is loaded with gurus, lousy with them. So is the United States. We just call them doctors.

We turn to them for direction and we listen for their divine wisdom, even when it contradicts our own. We may feel fine but still take a daily aspirin because a doctor says everyone over a certain age should. Or we may submit to invasive tests without asking the reason because we doubt our ability to understand the doctor's sophisticated thinking. We don't even ask; we just accept.

One afternoon in Pondicherry, I dropped into a comfy chair in a coffee house. Within minutes, an Englishman dropped into the chair beside me and dropped into conversation as if we were continuing one we started long ago, as if we'd known each other forever or that we would.

He was older than me, by ten or fifteen years, and the design on his T-shirt was faded and the cotton so soft I could see how it felt. He'd studied in Boulder and painted in London and spoke to me as if I were the only person in the café or maybe the only person in India. His kindness was that focused, that uncluttered, and his attention complete.

He asked how many times I'd been to India and I told him this was my first. He'd been too many times to count, traveling back and forth again and again over the previous twenty years.

"What keeps you coming back?" I asked.

"In the beginning, it was different gurus."

"There are a lot of them," I said.

"Yeah," he laughed. "And you know, it doesn't really matter who the guru is or what their teaching is. It's just about sitting in the presence of love. These gurus give unconditional love and that's where the magic is."

Later that afternoon, I relayed the conversation to Mitra and talked to her about all the gurus, all the different ideas and what held them all together.

"Yes," she said. "Do you know what *guru* means? It means 'Gee, you are you.'"

"Gee, you are you," I repeated. "That's genius."

It's true. After looking back on my crazy yearlong search for an answer to my medical woes—and after hearing from countless others who have been through similar painful experiences of diagnoses, misdiagnoses, *lack* of sufficient diagnoses, you name it—I've come to realize that only one thing counts. In a world filled with experts ready to give advice—medical, spiritual and any other kind—it's not the expert who matters as much as the person on the other side of the equation. Gee, you *are* you, and what are you going to do with the expert advice? How are you going to measure it and evaluate it against your own experience, hopes and dreams? And then, what are *you* going to do with it?

Each of us is our own expert, our own guru, capable of creating our own lives.

# AFTERWORD

Diagnosed or misdiagnosed—it's sometimes hard to tell which is which, and in retrospect, I was hoping to avoid them both. At the beginning of this journey, I wanted the tingling to go away, but I didn't want a medical expert to identify an illness or anything wrong with me. At the same time, I didn't want that expert to miss it if something was wrong. So I stumbled forward, going from doctor to doctor to doctor, hearing varied and conflicting theories.

At some point, when I started to see the humor in my tour of the American medical landscape, I could laugh at the lengths I traveled and the list of diagnoses endured. I had been diagnosed and diagnosed and diagnosed, from the time I was a kid all the way into my forties. I was *Miss* Diagnosed. If there was a crown, I could have worn it. I'd earned it.

And as I came to see the humor, I also saw something else: that the line between diagnosed and misdiagnosed is not always clear. The two are not mutually exclusive and neither a diagnosis nor a misdiagnosis can be exhaustive in describing the human body. A diagnosis can correctly identify a small piece of the puzzle while missing the big picture. (It was true I had vitamin deficiencies, but why?) And a mistake can correctly carve out a broad outline without catching the relevant detail. (One doctor said I had a leaky gut but failed to identify gluten as its cause.)

Ultimately, Dr. Desai was able to see a more complete story than the other doctors, and she was able to devise a plan that worked for me. A plan that worked with me. Certainly, she was able to do this because she's a great doctor trained in two medical traditions—Western and Ayurvedic—so she has her own system of checks and balances, of examining and reexamining from multiple angles. And she was able to devise a plan for me because, by the time I saw her, through trial and error, I knew what I wanted. I knew my goal, how I wanted to work with a doctor and how engaged I wanted to be in my own treatment.

In the United States, nearly 400,000 primary care physicians practice medicine and another 440,000 serve as specialists. All of them have expertise—no question—and they can run tests, ask questions and make diagnoses. None of them can know exactly what the patient wants, however, if the patient doesn't know.

I hope that none of you gets sick, that you don't have one day with some inexplicable symptom or confusing illness. That said, if you do have to go to a doctor, I hope you receive the care and results you want. And I think your chances of getting both increase dramatically if you walk into a doctor's office prepared.

Knowing your own preferences and desired outcomes can help, so here's a list of questions to get you started.

## BEFORE YOU SEE A DOCTOR...

Ask yourself what's going on in your body, be specific in your answers and stop to write it all down. Don't judge the answer and don't try to sort out the reason. Just identify what's happening. If, for example, you are tired, ask yourself:

- Is it a drowsiness like you want to sleep?
- Or a physical exhaustion, like you need to sit down?
- Do you feel better in the morning or the afternoon or at night?
- After a meal? Or when you haven't eaten?
- Is it exhaustion every day? Or specific days?

When you have a clear picture of what's bothering you, ask yourself what you would like to happen. What's the ideal outcome? Maybe the answer is obvious, like "I want to feel energized for a full sixteen hours a day." Or maybe it's less specific, like "I want to know when I'll have energy and when I'll feel tired so I can plan my days better." Maybe it's more fundamental: "I want to understand why I am tired so I can fix it."

With a picture of the perfect resolution, ask yourself what you're willing to do to get there. For example, most of us are willing to brush our teeth to avoid tooth decay. To resolve your symptoms, ask yourself whether are you willing to do the following:

- Change your diet? Your exercise routine?
- Adjust your sleep patterns?
- Take active steps to reduce stress?
- Go to physical therapy?
- Take medication? Swallow a pill daily? Inject yourself, if needed?
- Undergo surgery?

## DETERMINING TREATMENT

- Are you willing to ask questions until you understand what a doctor's telling you, in order to ensure that you are getting the right diagnosis and treatment, and that your health needs are being met?
- Are you willing to seek second, third and fourth opinions, if necessary?
- Is there a dollar amount over which you would pay no more for treatment?
- What factors will make you feel most comfortable with the doctor and most confident in her proposed treatment plan?
- Do you care if your doctor likes you or asks for your input or opinion? Do you need to like your doctor?
- What factors matter to you in terms of a finding the right doctor? What kind of qualifications, skills or background are you looking for in a doctor? How will those help you?

## QUESTIONS TO ASK YOUR DOCTOR

- How much time do we have together?
- Have you looked at my medical history, and are there any parts that seem unclear or questions I can answer for you?
- How do you like to work with your patients?
- Among your peers or colleagues, are you considered aggressive or conservative in the way you treat illness?
- Are you considered quick to order tests and treatments? Or more cautious?

- If I have questions, where do I go and whom do I ask for answers? How quickly can I expect an answer to my questions?
- It's important that I understand the reason for any test, treatment or medication. Will you work with me to make sure I understand?
- Could you tell me how you think about diet, exercise and other lifestyle choices as factors in health or healing? And where do pharmaceuticals fit into that picture?
- Are you a consultant or on the payroll of any pharmaceutical or medical equipment companies?

Then tell your doctor what you learned when you asked yourself the initial questions about your symptoms and desired outcomes, and ask if he or she can help you with that.

## QUESTIONS TO ASK BEFORE ANY MEDICAL TEST

- What's the reason for the test? What will it tell us? What will it rule out? And what will it rule in?
- How will the results of the test affect what we do next? (And if the answer is "not at all," skip the test.)
- How would we proceed if I don't want this test?
- What will it cost?
- Is this covered under my insurance plan and will having this test affect my premium?
- How long have you been using this test? What's your experience with it?
- How reliable are the results of this test?

- Is there another way to find the same information? A less expensive, less invasive and equally accurate test to consider?
- What are the possible adverse reactions to this test? How common are they?

## QUESTIONS TO ASK YOURSELF AFTER ANY MEDICAL TEST

- Do you want to be alone when you hear the results? Or would you prefer to have someone with you?
- And what role would you like them to play? Notetaker? Skeptic? Silent emotional supporter?

## QUESTIONS TO ASK THE DOCTOR AFTER A MEDICAL TEST

- What are the results? What do they lead you to believe?
- What else could cause the same results?
- Are there other ways to read this test?
- Is there another way to test the accuracy of this result?

## QUESTIONS ABOUT DRUGS AND DRUG TREATMENTS

- How long has this drug been on the market?
- What is it intended to do? How does it work?
- What are the common adverse effects? And the less common?
- How does it interact with other medications or supplements I'm taking?

- How frequently have you prescribed this medication? What results have you seen?
- What else do you know about this drug?
- What will it cost me?
- Are there alternatives, and what are the pros and cons of each?

# THE GOODS ON GLUTEN

Gluten is a protein found in wheat, barley, rye and other grains. It's the glue that holds dough together, allows it to rise, hold its shape and have a somewhat chewy texture when baked. Gluten's the thing that gives grief to anyone with celiac disease or a nonceliac gluten sensitivity. And surprisingly, it's also the specific part of really common grains that no one can digest.

Dr. Michael Marsh began studying the stuff more than thirty years ago. A British physician, Marsh has published hundreds of peer-reviewed papers and three books on the topic, and he lends his name to the classification system that doctors uses to identify symptoms of gluten sensitivity—Marsh I, Marsh II and Marsh III. Another world-renowned specialist, Dr. Alessio Fasano, founded and runs the University of Maryland Center for Celiac Research. Both doctors say that humans cannot digest gluten—that none of us has the enzymes to get the job done.

For many people though, it's not a problem. Gluten simply passes through and the body eliminates it without any drama.

The rest of us, however, are not so lucky. We have "gluten sensitivity," which means that our immune system—the army of white blood cells and other warriors designed to protect us—gets called to action when it encounters gluten. The immune system determines friend from foe, self from other, and 70 percent of this decision making occurs in the digestive tract. This long line of coordinated body parts forms an assembly line that runs from the mouth through the esophagus, stomach and intestines. More so than the skin, which interacts with the environment, the digestive tract offers the greatest interface between self and other. As food (which starts as "other") travels through the body, the digestive system works to break it down, and break it down further, while also sorting the molecules we need from the ones we don't. Ideally, the molecules that fuel us become so small through the process that they can pass through the intestine and into the bloodstream and be accepted as "self." Molecules we don't need and can't use are sent on their way.

This process goes off the rails for folks who can't tolerate gluten. For me, and others like me—up to 30 percent of the population by some calculations—my genetic code sounds the alarm when gluten is involved. For people with celiac disease or nonceliac gluten sensitivity, when gluten comes into contact with the lining of the intestine, it triggers an inflammatory response. The body reacts as if an invader were trying to get in. It creates inflammation and if the inflammation is consistent—as it would be in someone who doesn't know they're sensitive and eats wheat at every meal—the intestinal wall becomes irritated and starts breaking down. The tiny gaps that sit between cells and are supposed to let only the smallest and most useful molecules pass out of the intestine and into the bloodstream become enlarged. All of sudden, the tiny gaps are large gaps, and the indigestible gluten particles slip through. Once gluten hitches a ride on the bloodstream, it can wreak havoc anywhere in the body. Wherever it goes, it can trigger an immune response. That response—the inflammation—could be in the joints, or on the skin, anywhere really—which is why gluten sensitivity can manifest in so many ways. Here are some of them:

- Aching joints
- Anemia
- Depression
- Eczema
- Exhaustion
- Headaches
- Irritability or mood swings
- Nutritional deficiencies
- Osteoporosis
- Peripheral neuropathy
- Skin rashes
- Weight loss or weight gain

It's also why gluten sensitivity can be a tricky thing to diagnose. A patient with a skin condition may go to a dermatologist, who isn't thinking about anything starting in the belly. Same for a neurologist presented with a patient with peripheral neuropathy (tingling in the fingertips or toes).

Speaking at a recent Gluten Summit, David Perlmutter, a neurologist and the author of *Grain Brain*, compared the problem to firefighters who focus on the wrong danger. "Gluten sensitivity is the fire," Perlmutter said. "Drugs can treat the smoke but gluten sensitivity is the fire."

But here's the good news: treatment is simple and the cure can be complete.

For those of us with a genetic disposition, gluten triggers an immune response that over time can cause intestinal permeability, or "leaky gut." That permeability is what allows gluten to create inflammation beyond the digestive tract. Take away the trigger though, and there is no immune response, and eventually, the gut can heal. But you have to take away the trigger all the time. As long as gluten continues to irritate the lining of the intestine, that tissue cannot repair itself. (Picture a scab that keeps getting scratched. Or maybe a pair of lungs that belong to a smoker—as long as he keeps smoking, each cigarette adds insult to injury, and the lungs continue to suffer.)

Once gluten is eliminated from the diet, it may take a while, but the long-irritated tissue can settle down and repair itself, which in turn can relieve the symptoms. It may not be overnight and going to zero tolerance can be difficult, but in my experience, it's worth it and worth knowing how to avoid gluten completely.

Beyond the obvious gluten-filled foods like cookies, cakes, breads and cereals, gluten creeps its way into almost everything in a box, bag or bottle in a grocery store. Few people toss flour into a salad dressing or tomato sauce when they're cooking at home, but many store-bought bottles include gluten as a thickener. Gluten shows up as binders in salamis, fermenting agents in soy products and stabilizers in ice creams. It's in chewing gum, chocolate bars and malted-milk balls. And packaging doesn't list gluten in the ingredients because often gluten is inside another ingredient, not added independently. The only way to avoid it with packaged foods is to look for the big "GF" or "Gluten-Free" label. Luckily, in 2013, the Food and Drug Administration issued rules to standardize the labeling so that "GF" means the same thing everywhere.

## FINDING OUT IF GLUTEN IS A PROBLEM FOR YOU

With unexplained symptoms or runaway inflammation, gluten could be the culprit. To find out for sure, doctors can suggest a blood test, a stool test, an intestinal biopsy or an elimination diet. Dr. Peter Green, director of the Celiac Disease Center at Columbia University and author of *Celiac Disease: A Hidden Epidemic*, says it this way, "Anyone who has symptoms brought on by the ingestion of gluten that are relieved by its removal from the diet can be called gluten intolerant."

To find out if that's the case, anyone can do an elimination diet. Some people worry about what they might lose in the process but Dr. Mark Hyman, a leading thinker in integrative medicine, puts those fears to rest this way: "Gluten is not an essential nutrient."

In the beginning, however, going gluten-free may be daunting. For a while, I was so afraid of hidden gluten, I cooked every meal at home. That no longer seems necessary. Most restaurants, from high-end chefs like Thomas Keller to low-budget burrito joints like Chipotle, can accommodate a gluten-free diet. And most servers know what I mean when I say, "I have a gluten thing."

To learn which restaurants can serve people with celiac disease or with gluten sensitivity, which recipes will work, and which grocery store brands are safe, there are plenty of resources online, including the following:

www.celiaccentral.org
www.celiac.com
www.csaceliacs.info
www.gluten.net
www.glutenfreeliving.com
www.glutenfreewatchdog.org

The Paleo diet is also gluten-free, so anything Paleo fits the bill.

There are apps for your phone, dozens of cookbooks and hundreds of blogs that will send you gluten-free recipes or coupons for GF goods, or both, every day. A gluten-free life may seem challenging, but it's really not. And if gluten creates any chronic symptoms, going gluten-free beats the alternative.

And to find a doctor who can help you sort it out, integrated or functional medical specialists are one way to go. You can search for doctors near you at the following:

www.functionalmedicine.org
www.integrativemedicine.arizona.edu

All of us, I believe, can take charge of our health. It's helpful to have a trained professional working with us and giving us information and options. And some of us have more obstacles in our path than others, but all of us can become informed, make our own choices and do the best we can for ourselves.

I wish all of you all your very best health!

# SUGGESTED READING

Amen, Daniel G. *Change Your Brain, Change Your Life: The Breakthrough Program for Conquering Anxiety, Depression, Obsessiveness, Anger, and Impulsiveness*. New York: Times Books, 2000.

Boroch, Ann. *Healing Multiple Sclerosis: Diet, Detox & Nutritional Makeover for Total Recovery*. Los Angeles: Quintessential Healing, 2007.

Chopra, Deepak. *Perfect Health*. New York: Bantam, 1990.

Chodron, Pema. *When Things Fall Apart: Heart Advice for Difficult Times*. Boston: Shambhalam, 1997.

Cordain, Loren. *The Paleo Diet: Lose Weight and Get Healthy by Eating the Food You Were Designed to Eat*. New York: Wiley, 2002.

Doidge, Norman. *The Brain That Changes Itself: Stories of Personal Triumph from the Frontiers of Brain Science*. New York: Viking, 2007.

Green, Peter H. R., and Rory Jones. *Celiac Disease: A Hidden Epidemic*. New York: HarperCollins, 2006.

Groopman, Jerome E. *How Doctors Think*. Boston: Houghton Mifflin, 2007.

Hyman, Mark. *The UltraMind Solution: Fix Your Broken Brain by*

*Healing Your Body First—The Simple Way to Defeat Depression, Overcome Anxiety and Sharpen Your Mind*. New York: Scribner, 2008.

Kabat-Zinn, Jon. *Full Catastrophe Living: Using the Wisdom of Your Body and Mind to Face Stress, Pain, and Illness*. New York: Dell, 1991.

Mate, Gabor. *When the Body Says No: Understanding the Stress-Disease Connection*. Hoboken, NJ: Wiley, 2003.

Moynihan, Ray, and Alan Cassels. *Selling Sickness: How the World's Biggest Pharmaceutical Companies Are Turning Us All into Patients*. New York: Nation Books, 2005.

Mullin, Gerard E., and Kathie Madonna Swift. *The Inside Tract: Your Good Gut Guide to Great Digestive Health*. New York: Rodale, 2011.

Perlmutter, David, and Kristin Loberg. *Grain Brain: The Surprising Truth about Wheat, Carbs, and Sugar—Your Brain's Silent Killers*. New York: Little, Brown, 2013.

Siegel, Daniel J. *Mindsight: The New Science of Personal Transformation*. New York: Bantam Books, 2010.

Wahls, Terry. *The Wahls Protocol: How I Beat Progressive MS Using Paleo Principles and Functional Medicine*. New York: Penguin, 2014.

Weil, Andrew. *Health and Healing*, rev. ed. Boston: Houghton Mifflin, 1988.

Welch, H. Gilbert, Lisa Schwartz, and Steve Woloshin. *Overdiagnosed: Making People Sick in the Pursuit of Health*. Boston: Beacon Press, 2011.

# ACKNOWLEDGMENTS

I am grateful for all my friends and family who held my hand, kept me laughing and loved me as I bounced from doctor to doctor. My dad, Dawn and Andrei Gorlitsky, Lisa Smith, Joe Mahoney, Jeremy Shaver, Mitra Tredway, Wayne Tisdale and of course, my constant companion, Riley, all cheered me on and cheered me up every step of the way.

Doctors and healers of all kinds taught me about healing and offered their wisdom and generosity in guiding me to a healthier version of me. I'm grateful for Anthony Fulker, Stuart Gross, Myron MacDonald, Philippe Souvestre, Nita Desai and Orianne Evans.

Thank you to Peter Trachtenberg, who was the first person to read any of my pages and who told me to keep going. I took his advice and found in Denver a truly supportive writing community at the Lighthouse Writers Workshop. I'm thankful for Lighthouse founders Andrea Dupree and Michael Henry, and all the great writers who read my work and gave me their feedback and encouragement: Paula Altschuler, Regina Drexler, Suzanne Finney, Jay Kenney, Betsy Leighton, Cheryl Strayed and Paula Younger.

My agent, Laura Yorke, read and liked my proposal and made sure it found its way to a wonderful editor. And my editor at Sourcebooks, Stephanie Bowen, read closely enough to know me and guided my story with a sure and gentle hand. *Misdiagnosed* is a much better book because of her insight. Thank you.

# ABOUT THE AUTHOR

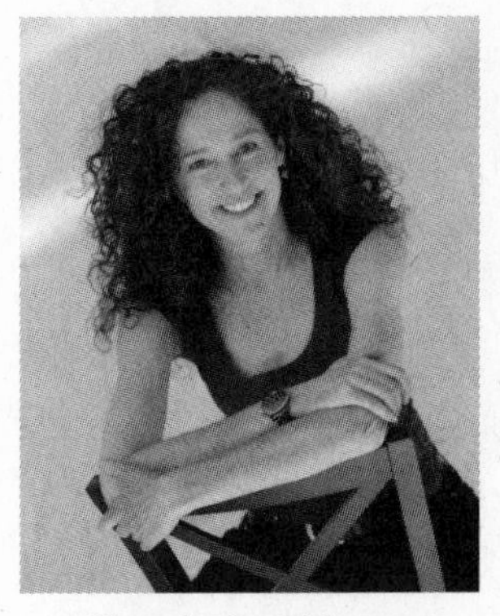

Photo by Joe Mahoney

Jody Berger is a freelance journalist and certified holistic health coach. She was a reporter for *ESPN* magazine for five years, helping to shape the way it covered extreme sports, and she freelanced for *Self, Teen People, Harper's Bazaar* and others. Subsequently, she became a reporter for *Rocky Mountain News*, where she led the editorial teams at the Salt Lake City, Athens and Turin Olympic Games. She was awarded the prestigious Knight Fellowship at Stanford University, and graduated from the Institute for Integrative Nutrition. She lives in Denver, Colorado, and blogs at jody-berger.com.